121

Cover Design by Vishalklair
Book Edited by Cedric Mixon & Kesha Burns
Resources:
The Holy Bible, NKJ, NIV, NLT ©1984, Thomas Nelson, Inc.
Drugs in Modern Society: Charles R. Carroll. Alcohol Problems & Alcoholism: James E. Royce
Excerpts taken from "Man By the Side of the Road", by Dr. Ronald L. Bobo Sr.

For information:
Kobalt Books, P.O. Box 1062, Bala Cynwyd, PA 19004
Printed in the U.S.A
www.kobaltbooks.com

Published by Kobalt Books L.L.C.
An original publication of Kobalt Books L.L.C.

121

OVERCOMING DRUG ADDICTION BY FAITH

by
BURTON BARR JR.

KOBALT BOOKS

Contents

Acknowledgements

———— † ————

There are so many people that God has brought into my life that I am truly grateful for. Many of them are part of my church family at West Side Missionary Baptist Church in St. Louis, Missouri. I thank God for all of them. I thank God for my former pastor, Dr. Ronald L. Bobo, Sr. and his lovely wife, Darlean. I thank God for my new pastor, Rev. Charles H.N. Bobo and his wife Michelle. I thank God for my friend, Dr. Rosalind P. Denson. She taught me the meaning of integrity.

I am thankful for my wife, Charlotte, my daughter, Andrea, my son, Markus and my grandchildren. They are the pride of my life. I am thankful for my family members. I love them all.

I thank God for the precious memories of five special people: my sister, Shirley Jones, my niece, Christine Sumuel, my cousin, Gary Jones, and my very dear friends, Sandy Bailey and Rev. Carl Smith who all transitioned from this life in the past year. May they rest in paradise. I also thank God for the life of a young lady that I never met. Her name is Deshaye Collins and her story inspired me to write this book.

Burton Barr Jr.

This book is dedicated to my father, Rev. Burton Barr, Sr. I learned so much from him. When I was going through my darkest hours because of my addiction, he never gave up on me. He encouraged me and told me to trust in the Lord. Dad was killed in 1988, but sometimes I hear those words of wisdom that he shared with me. I love you Dad.

Foreword

I have known Reverend Burton Barr, Jr. for over 20 years as church member, colleague and valued staff member at a large, metropolitan church, where I am privileged to serve as the Associate Pastor, Chief of Staff, and Minister of Congregational Care and Counseling. Over time, he has become a trusted brother and friend.

Burton is a master storyteller whose humor and authenticity draw you into his message. The entire church looked forward to hearing about his escapades with his associates. He was real about the pain of addiction, for both the people with addictions and their loved ones. After laughing, smiling, and sometimes wiping away tears, we could not dismiss these unique individuals with a derogatory label or self-righteously turn away — for we could see our own human frailties and need for a Savior. Burton's messages were always full of the hope of God's power to protect, heal, and deliver.

Burton's dedication to help the weary, wounded and sad through prison ministry has resulted in people being saved, baptized, delivered, rededicated, or reconciled with families. You might wonder, however, what his prison ministry has to do with addiction and recovery. Did you know that of 2.3 million U.S. inmates, 1.5 million suffer from substance abuse addiction? Alcohol and other drugs are significant factors in all crimes, including 78% of violent crimes, 83% of property crimes and 77% of public order, immigration, weapons offenses, and probation and parole violations (Behind Bars 11, Substances Abuse and America's Prison Population).

So, as Burton ministered to the prison population, he often ministered to those with a history of substance abuse. His work was not just behind bars, but he also established an aftercare program to assist inmates upon release and started an Angel Tree Program to provide gifts to the children of inmates at Christmas.

Burton's strong and abiding faith in God though, began with seeds planted by a Christian father and was forged in the fires of tribulation and trials, misery, and the anguish of addiction. Caught up in a lifestyle that wrecked relationships, produced financial devastation and led him to the brink of death, he managed to hold on to the hope that God would help him. Many preachers were born under circumstances that looked sterile and barren, but God, using Burton, had the last word.

This book is for the families and friends of those who are addicted: who have walked floors, cleaned up messes, raised abandoned children, suffered thefts and betrayal and yet still love their "Bub," by whatever name. It will help give insight into what people with addiction are going through and "why they just won't quit."

It is for those who minister to the addicted and want greater understanding of these precious souls for whom God sent His Son to die.

It is for the people who are entangled and wonder if there is a way out, if God hears their cries, and if He will even bother to answer.

Burton has written this insightful and encouraging book to help people understand what they are signing up for when they experiment with drugs, to help families and loved ones cope with the pain of addiction, and to share the Good News that God has a plan for our lives. He is a God of amazing, unconditional, unmerited love; and He has all power to save, heal, and deliver.

- Rev. Rosalind P. Denson Ph.D

Burton Barr Jr.

Introduction

✝

During the height of my drug addiction, my father came to me one day. He didn't start preaching at me and telling me that I needed to quit. He didn't talk about the hurt and the pain that I was causing my family. He didn't tell me about the damage that I was doing to myself. He just opened his Bible to a certain scripture. He gave it to me and told me to read that scripture every morning before I left home. The scripture was **Psalms 121**. It says:

I will lift up my eyes to the hills-
From whence comes my help.

My help comes from the Lord,
Who made heaven and earth.

He will not allow your foot to be moved;
He who keeps you will not slumber.

Behold, He who keeps Israel
Shall neither slumber nor sleep.

The Lord is your keeper;
The Lord is your shade at your right hand.

The sun shall not strike you by day'
Nor the moon by night.

The Lord shall preserve you from all evil;
He shall preserve your soul.

The Lord shall preserve your going out
and your coming in from this time forth,
and even forever more.

I read that scripture every morning, no matter how drunk or high I was. Sometimes, I was so high, I couldn't see the words. So I had my lady friend or whoever was in my house read it to me. That was my connection to God. I was a criminal and a dope fiend, but the words in that scripture comforted me and gave me peace.

I was talking to my father one day. I think he knew I was in trouble. He said, "Son, whenever you need help, just look to the hills and call on the Lord." There are no hills on the west side of Chicago, but I knew what he meant.

This book is about addictions and how they disrupt the lives of so many people. I will talk about some of the experiences that I had and what happened to some of the people that I knew. Some of the names have been changed, but their stories are true. The subtitle of this book is, "Overcoming Drug Addiction By Faith." The Bible says, "Faith without works is dead." (James 2:26) By faith, we can trust God to deliver us from our addiction. However, there are some things that we must do.

It doesn't matter what you are going through right now. You may have been knocked down so many times, you are afraid to get up again. I speak from experience when I say; you don't have to live like that. What inspired me to change my life was the scripture my father told me to read every day when I was struggling, Psalms **121**.

Burton Barr Jr.

121 Mission Statement
*"To encourage and inspire an addict to get sober today --
For at least one addict on this planet to turn away from the
drugs and choose life instead of death. Live, young king.
Live, young queen..."*

In Too Deep

———————— † ————————

1969. West-side Chicago. I was 20 years old and snorting a drug they called "Duji" with my friends B.B., Ronnie and Tadpole. That was my introduction to the game -- the dope game. Little did I know that Duji was actually heroin and I'd soon find out what it feels like to "take the needle." My virgin-veins had never been sullied until one dreadful Friday night that I'll never forget.

B.B., Ronnie and Tadpole came by my house to hang out, but instead of bringing the usual marijuana and alcohol, they came with makeshift syringes filled with Duji. B.B. said, "I brought something but this time, we're gonna shoot it!" Not interested, I told them to just set mine aside and I'll snort my portion later. Ronnie said, "Nah, you don't understand. We're shooting ours and you're gonna shoot it to!" I didn't realize it, but B.B. and Ronnie came up to me from behind while Tadpole approached with the needle. "Sorry Bub, I know this is the only way I can get you to try it." I fought them with everything in me but eventually, the needle found its way into my arm. "Hey, you need to quit moving before the needle breaks in your arm," said Ronnie. All I could think about was locating my gun and killing everyone in this room when this is all over. Suddenly, a feeling of euphoria came over me. The heroin had become one with my system and my rage, worries, sadness, loneliness, and insecurities were all replaced with peace.

The first time I shot heroin, I thought it was the best thing ever. I had tried other drugs, such as weed, reds, trees, acid, and booze but nothing gave me that mellow feeling like heroin. Like the great songstress Sade says, "it's never as good as the first time." Although I was addicted to heroin, I was able to leave it alone for periods of time. The problem was, I always came back.

With cocaine, I was hooked the first time. By the time I was shooting cocaine with a needle, I was officially a slave to the next high – many times, checking my pockets to see how much money I had so I could buy some more even while the needle was still in my arm.

My addiction cost me a lot, both financially and relationally. I probably spent more than $200,000 during my 22-plus year addiction. All of my criminal activity was brought on because of my addiction. Most of my crimes were retail theft or some type of check schemes.

All of us have made mistakes in our lives. You, or someone that you know, might be suffering the consequences that bad choices bring. I know, because I've made more than my share of them as well. I've been addicted to heroin, cocaine, alcohol, crack, marijuana, and PCP. I thank God for sending a preacher to the prison one day. He told me that I didn't have to let where I am, dictate who I am.

Some people who were familiar with my past addictions asked me how I was able to get off drugs. Some of them wanted me to talk to their family members or loved ones who are addicted, seeing as how my addictions lasted more than 22 years. I was able to stay clean for periods of time during those years but scripture tells us, *"like a dog returns to his own vomit, a fool repeats his folly."* (Proverbs 26:11)

During my addiction, I thought I was only hurting myself. Nothing was further from the truth. The pain and anguish that is felt by family members and loved ones is overwhelming and unbearable.

I knew I was in too deep when I started running con games on family members who loved me. I was addicted to all types of drugs, including alcohol and I used crime to fund it all.

The drugs didn't replace anything. I just seemed to be chasing something that wasn't there. I lost friends because of my addiction. It strained the relationship with a lot of my family members because they couldn't trust me. My marriage failed because I chose drugs over family.

I was told that people get high for one of two

reasons: To feel good, or not to feel. I got high for both reasons. I was trying to escape reality. The thing that most people don't realize is, no one can help an addict until he or she really wants help. An addict will not seek or accept help until he or she really wants to quit. This does not just apply to drugs; it applies to all forms of addiction.

I knew that I could die because of drugs. After all, I had overdosed several times but overdose is not the only way that people die because of drugs. I was robbed at gunpoint several times on my way in, or on my way out of drug houses.

I used to think being locked up was just an occupational hazard. It came with the territory. Looking back, I think the police were not arresting me; instead they were rescuing me from myself. There is absolutely nothing that I miss about that life. I do, however, miss some of the people that I knew. What a lot of people don't know is that hidden beneath all the hurt, pain and shame of addiction, there's a beautiful man or woman that the world either never knew existed or has long forgotten. There's a diamond in that rough. There's a butterfly in that cocoon. There's an angel in all that darkness.

I never got to a point where I didn't want to live, but I did get to a point where I knew I could die. Surprisingly, I didn't care. Hopelessness is the worst feeling there is and it had surrounded me. I'd given up on ever becoming anything or being truly happy. What I now know is that God was with me when I was living that hoodlum lifestyle. That's the only way I could've possibly survived the shootings, stabbings, overdoses, robberies and prison.

When I was in prison, a prison ministry preacher named Rev. Jerry Hodges came to my cell block one day. He said, "Hey my brother. Why don't you come to the bible study tonight? God has a word for you." I went that night and my life has never been the same.

God delivered me from a life of drugs and crime. I continue walking in my deliverance through faith in Him and remembering where He brought me from. The triggers that I had, no longer influence me but there are situations that I don't put myself in anymore. Like the saying goes, "a man has got to know his limitations." I've had several support groups and people that I could talk to to help me stay on the right track. Some are family members. Some are church members. Some are friends.

I was walking around the prison yard one day when I heard God say, "Just like I sent Rev. Hodges to the prison to rescue you, I will send you back to the prisons to rescue others." My purpose is to encourage the men and women who are in prison by letting them know that they don't have to let where they are, dictate who they are. That is why God created me. That is why He allowed me to go through the things that I went through.

When I preach or teach at various jails and prisons, I tell inmates, "There are people who will not listen to me, but they will listen to you. You have to reach out to your families and friends so they won't end up in prison, or worse."

My testimony allowed me to reach people that society had thrown away and I believe God spoke to me through Rev. Hodges. If I had not accepted the ministry that He called me to, I believe a lot of people whose lives were changed because of our ministry would have been lost, and I would be held accountable. I believe that people who never overcome their addictions will eventually end up in prison or suffer an early death. That is what my eyes have seen.

The opening words to one of Rick Warren's books is, "It's not about you." God sometimes allows us to go through situations so we can bless others who are going through the same situations. Notice, I said God *allows* us, not God *makes* us. God gives us free will to choose our paths. If we realize we have chosen the wrong path and turn around, God will then use us to warn others not to continue on that path. That is what I do in the prisons. That is what I do when I talk to drug addicts, but in the words of Rick Warren, "It's not about me." God called me to this ministry. It is all about Him.

I have learned to trust God in all things. I know He

has a plan for my life. Considering how far down I fell when I hit "rock bottom", some of the things that God has done in my life completely blows my mind. I know beyond a shadow of a doubt that it is He, who is performing all these miracles in my life. The good news is, He can do the same for you! By the grace of God, I have regained the trust and respect of my family and friends.

Rev. Hodges gave me the most powerful message more than 30 years ago, "No matter what you've done, no matter what you've become, God still loves you." My advice to people who are trying to get and stay clean is something that my father once told me, "If you slip and fall down, get up and keep stepping. If you fall down again, get up again. If you keep falling down, keep getting up."

Being clean all these years is priceless but I still bear scars from my addiction. When people start, they often think it's no big deal. They think that they can handle it. Not knowing that drugs are like quick sand, they fail to realize the trouble they're in until it's too late. I'm here to tell you that if God can deliver me from my addictions, He can deliver you from yours too.

I believe God loves us regardless of what we have done. The Bible is full of stories about God's love, grace and redeeming power but the stories didn't end in Biblical times. If you don't believe it, just look at me. I was tired of heroin and the effect that my addiction was having on me, my family, my friends and everyone that cared about me. I wanted to quit, but I couldn't.

One night, I went on my back porch and threw my syringe over the banister into the alley. "I quit!" I thought the problem was solved and my addictions were finally defeated. I was so proud of myself. Imagine the disgust I had in myself when just a few hours later, I was crawling around that dark, dirty, filthy alley on my hand and knees with a cigarette lighter, trying to find that same needle and syringe. Look at what I had become. I was in too deep. I was a lost sheep. I was an addict. I was a dope fiend.

I can't explain why someone would go back to a drug that he or she knows could be detrimental to their life. Maybe I wanted to try to get that feeling that I had the first time I shot up. Maybe I thought I could handle it and wanted to do it just once or twice more. Or maybe, that time, I was trying to fill a void in my life.

When I moved to St. Louis, I asked one of my cousins for directions somewhere. He told me that the quickest way was to take the shortcut through Forest Park. For those of you who are not familiar with St. Louis, Forest Park is a large park with lots of attractions, including the St. Louis Zoo.

As I was driving through the park, I noticed that there were a lot of turns, curves, and side roads in there. It seemed like every turn that I made was the wrong turn and every road that I took was the wrong road. I had gotten to the point that I didn't care what street I came out on, I just wanted out of that park!

I started praying and begging God to get me out. I got so scared, I started praying one of those, "I ain't gonna do it no more" prayers. I said, "Lord, if you will just get me out of this park, I promise that I will never set foot in here again." Some of you all know the kind of prayer that I am talking about, the "I ain't gonna do it no more" prayers.

When I finally found my way out of Forest Park that day, I swore that I would never drive through there again. But some time later, I was driving around in the area. And I started looking at that park. Then I started thinking to myself, "I know I got lost when I was in there before, but it wasn't *all* bad. You know, it really *is* a beautiful park and is kind of peaceful in there. Maybe I got lost because I went too far." I got in too deep.

I decided to go back into Forest Park and just stay on a road where I can still see the streets. I was driving along and enjoying the scenery when all of a sudden, the road that I was traveling on took a sharp turn. I couldn't see the street anymore and I couldn't turn around because the road that I was traveling on was a one way street heading deeper and deeper into Forest Park.

Reminiscing can be a dangerous thing sometimes. You start thinking about the stuff you used to do and you say, "it wasn't *all* bad. I did have some good times back then. I just went too far. I got in too deep. I can do *some* of those things again." Before you know it, you're deep in your addiction again.

Coke Lies

— † —

Most of my crimes were either retail theft or theft by deception. I was working as a sales person at JC Penny. I had missed work while on a cocaine binge. When I ran out of drugs, I went to work so I could steal some more VCRs. I called my crime partner, Buck, to help get them out of the store.

I had heard that store security had been suspecting me for quite some time. I didn't care. I thought I was too smart for them. What I didn't know was, they had brought in a person whose only job was to watch me. They got me.

I had heard that if you wrote a bad check to a store, if they accepted partial payment on the check, they could not press charges. So, I would write a check for something that was priced at about $600.00. (In those days, it took almost two weeks for a check to return.)

After a day or two, I would go back to the store and give the manager a sob story. I would give him $50.00 or $100.00 and promise to pay the balance when I got paid. It worked every time! Days later, I was arrested for an unrelated case. I couldn't make bail and I couldn't get back to the stores with the partial payments.

A few weeks later, some detectives came to the jail and arrested me again. I thought that was the dumbest thing I had ever heard of. How can you arrest someone who's already in jail? It turned out that while I was in jail, stores in two other suburbs had pressed charges against me. So they added another $50,000 to my ransom, and moved me to a more secure section of the jail.

When I was in the marines, one of my crime partners and I sold kilos (called bricks) of marijuana. Most of our sales were legit, but sometimes we would prey on unsuspecting servicemen that were being discharged by packaging some grass from someone's lawn. We put about an ounce of real marijuana in a strategic place so they could test it. Years later, I sold fake heroin, cocaine and crack. Those were some very dangerous games. Those games could have cost me my life. A couple of times, they almost did.

I ran a lot of con games on people but the ones that bothered me most were the games that I played on my family. Actually, most of them were what I called, "coke lies". Addicts can easily fool their loved ones because they love them and want to believe them. Even when they think you are lying, they give you the benefit of the doubt. They really want to believe that this time, you're telling the truth.

Most of the men in my family were alcoholics at

some point in their lives, including my father, grandfather, uncles and cousins. I think it was the call from God that made my father get sober.

One night, I went to a drug house to buy a ten-dollar bag of heroin. Dealers served their customers through a first-floor window facing an alley. After making my purchase, I was walking to my car when I saw someone walking towards me. He pointed a gun at me and said, "Give it up?" I acted like I didn't know what he was talking about. He came closer and said, "Give me the dope!" That wasn't going to happen. I didn't have any more money.

I dropped the bag on the ground and put my foot on it so he couldn't see it. I told him that I had dropped the bag when I saw him coming because I thought he was the police. He cocked the gun and said, "I'm not going to tell you again." I took my foot off the bag so he could see it. I said, "There it is. I told you I dropped it."

I was hoping he would bend down to pick it up so I could kick him in his head but he told me to get in my car. I got in my car as fast as I could so I could run him over. When I looked up, he had disappeared! I was willing to die for a ten-dollar bag of heroin but more importantly, I was willing to take someone else's life because of it.

I made a lot of acquaintances during my drug years. When I decided to get clean, I knew I had to distance myself from them. I think about some of them from time to time, but I haven't seen or heard from most of them in years. I've heard of some who died as a result of the life. The drug/criminal lifestyle took the lives of most of my childhood friends: Red was found in a hotel room with his throat cut, Fuzzy was found in his bedroom with a needle in his arm and Butch died from an overdose. I know of some, who overcame their addictions. I led my good friend, Tadpole, to Christ during one of my visits to Chicago. He was clean for more than 15 years. We kept in touch over the years but unfortunately, he passed away in 2017. I don't know why God let me live when so many others died. Maybe it was because of the work He had for me to do. Perhaps all of this is connected to a divine purpose that He has over our lives. If God did it for me, He can do it for you too.

My father bought the two-family flat where I grew up in the early 1950s. We were the first black family in the neighborhood. When we moved in, the white families started moving out. It was a nice, quiet and peaceful neighborhood where everyone knew and looked out for each other. All that changed in the 80s.

Crack and gangs infiltrated city streets. As drug and gang activity moved in, businesses and hard-working residents moved out, but my father stood up to them. I used and sold drugs. When he found out, he didn't cut me any slack. My father would take to the streets and speak life to the addicts, prostitutes and anyone else that was lost. In doing so, he created a lot of enemies. One Saturday morning, dad was run down by a hit and run driver while crossing a street by his home. Witnesses said it looked like he was targeted. He died three days later.

Unfortunately, my father didn't live to see the change in my life but one thing I know with certainty, he never stopped praying for me. My biggest regret is the pain and embarrassment that I caused him.

I hurt and embarrassed my family many times with arrests and jail and prison sentences. They were hurt with their knowledge of my addictions but what I remember most was a letter that I got from my 15-year-old daughter when I was in prison. She lived in Detroit with her mother. When I got to the prison in Joliet, Illinois I wrote her a letter. Several weeks later, I received a return letter from her. She said, "Dad. Why is the only time I hear from you is when you are in jail?" Apparently, even my daughter had had enough of my little coke lies. She was tired of me telling her, "Daddy's gonna do better." She no longer believed my lies. No one did.

During the final years of my addiction, I stole from everyone, including the church. I found my father's tithes envelope one night and took the cash out of it. I found the church's check book and forged several checks. I was completely out of control. This was "rock bottom" for me.

Burton Barr Jr.

Stealing from the church was the one thing I said I would never do. Because of my addiction, I walked away from God and my calling but oddly enough, I never stopped believing in Him.

My first day of sobriety wasn't special. I'd had a lot of "first days" but after being clean for a month, I thought I could hang out with my old friends. It didn't work. I relapsed. After that, I was more determined than ever to stay clean. The first month felt good. After three months, I was doing well, but I knew that I needed help. I found it in my renewed relationship with God.

One of the things that helped me get there was the scripture my father told me to read every day when I was struggling with drugs. Psalms **121**.

Why Don't You Quit?

I love Jazz. I love listening to the sweet sounds of gifted artists like Miles Davis, Stanley Turrentine, Grover Washington Jr., Jimmy Smith and Wes Montgomery just to name a few. One of my favorite musicians is the legendary Gene "Jug" Ammons. The first time I'd ever heard of him was when I was in The Star Fire Lounge on Homan Avenue near Grenshaw Street in Chicago. The D.J. was playing a cut called "Ca' Purange (Jungle Soul)." I had never heard anyone play the tenor sax like that before. Sometime later, I heard other records of his, such as Angel Eyes and Canadian Sunset. I was an instant Gene Ammons fan.

Ammons had recently been released from prison after serving seven years of a 15-year sentence on narcotics charges. Shortly after his release, he put out a new album named, "The Boss Is Back." The number one tune on the album was a cut called, "The Jungle Boss." Although I liked that tune, I will never forget the time I heard Ammons play a cut that was recorded by Eddie Harris titled, "Why Don't You Quit?"

Like many jazz artists of the 50s and 60s, Ammons was believed to have been addicted to heroin. Even with all of his success in the music industry and his two stints in prison, he was unable to kick his habit. This is purely speculation on my part, but some of his friends and relatives, who probably meant well, kept asking him, "Why don't you quit?" Well, speaking from experience, that is easier said than done.

I was addicted to heroin and cocaine for more than twenty-two years. During that time there were so many friends, relatives and even law enforcement, who kept asking me that same question, "Why don't you quit?" I was never so tired of hearing any one question in my life. I can only imagine how tired Ammons was of hearing it. That might have been the reason he was able to play that song with so much feeling. Why don't you quit?

Since I have been clean and drug free, the number one question that I hear has gone from "Why don't you quit?" to "How did you quit?" People want to know how I overcame my drug addiction. After writing my first book, "The Hoodlum Preacher," some people have asked me if I was going to write a sequel, detailing step by step how to quit doing drugs. Well, I wish it were that easy but unfortunately it is not.

There are literally thousands, maybe even millions of people who are strung out on something; drugs, alcohol, cigarettes, gambling, pornography, etc. To those who are on the outside looking in, the solution seems simple but to those who are caught up in their various habits, it is a different story.

There are a lot of people who have been able to turn their lives around by using different methods. However, I can only tell you what worked for me and hundreds of other people that I know of. It was the power of God through Jesus Christ.

The problem is, people want to put God in a box. They think He only works in certain ways. The truth is, God works in many ways and through many people and programs, but that is not what we were taught in Sunday school. Therefore, we are always looking for the Damascus Road experience (Acts chapter 9), a miraculous delivery.

God has miraculously healed many people. Others had to go to the hospital or undergo surgery. Likewise, He has miraculously delivered a lot of people from drugs and alcohol, while others had to go to treatment centers. The truth is, God sometimes uses doctors, hospitals, treatment centers, 12-step programs, or the power of prayer to heal or deliver us from our situations. Sometimes, He even uses prison.

I don't know why He does what He does or why He works the way He chooses. When you get to heaven, you can ask Him for yourself, or maybe, He has already given us the answer. *"For My thoughts are not your thoughts, nor are your ways My ways, says the Lord. For as the heavens are higher than the earth, so are My ways higher than your ways, and My thoughts than your thoughts."* *(Isaiah 55:8-9)*

The story was told of a man who was trapped on his roof during a terrible flood. As the water rose dangerously high, a man came by in a row boat to rescue him. But the man refused to get in the boat. He said, "That's all right. God will save me." The water had risen even higher when someone in a helicopter came to his rescue. But again, the man refused help, saying, "That's all right. God will save me."

The water eventually rose above the man's head, and he drowned. When he arrived in heaven he was angry with God for allowing him to drown. He said, "Lord, why didn't you rescue me from that roof?" God said, "I tried. I sent a helicopter and a boat." God works in many ways.

I was not able to quit using drugs until I became brutally honest with myself and stopped trying to run games on people and accepted God's help, His way. I had gone to treatment centers several times before, but I never really gave it my all. Most of the time, I was just trying to appease someone or get out of trouble. I had gotten to the point that I realized that if I continued living that kind of life I would soon be dead or in some very serious trouble.

Besides that, I was hurting so many people that

loved me. My arms looked terrible. Because of the tracks, I wore long sleeve shirts or jackets all the time. My veins were getting so damaged it was getting harder and harder for me to get a hit. I had run con games on so many people, no one wanted to be around me, including other junkies. I was tired of going to jail. Boy, was I tired.

I had ripped off my father and aunt so many times; they couldn't even afford to buy food. I hated myself for what I had become and what I was doing to so many people but still, I could not quit.

One Sunday morning in November of 1991, I went to a drug house to get a one-and-one. This particular drug house ran a special on Sunday mornings from 9am till noon -- Buy one bag and get another one for half price. I was walking past a church after I had copped the heroin and cocaine. Somehow, I was able to hear the sermon that was being preached. It was the story of the prodigal son, also known as, the lost son. It is a parable that Jesus told one day and is recorded in the 15th chapter in the Gospel of St. Luke.

In it, Jesus said, *"There was a man who had two sons. The younger one said to his father, 'Father, give me my share of the estate.' So he divided his property between them."*

"Not long after that, the younger son got together all he had, set off for a distant country, and there

squandered his wealth in wild living. After he had spent everything, there was a severe famine in that whole country, and he began to be in need. So he went and hired himself out to a citizen of that country, who sent him to his fields to feed pigs. He longed to fill his stomach with the pods that the pigs were eating, but no one gave him anything."

"When he came to his senses, he said, 'How many of my father's hired servants have food to spare, and here I am starving to death! I will set out and go back to my father and say to him: Father, I have sinned against heaven and against you. I am no longer worthy to be called your son; Make me like one of your hired servants.' So he got up and went to his father."

"But while he was still a long way off, his father saw him and was filled with compassion for him; he ran to his son, threw his arms around him and kissed him.

"The son said to him, 'Father, I have sinned against heaven and against you. I am no longer worthy to be called your son."

"But the father said to his servants, 'Quick, bring the best robe and put it on him. Put a ring on his finger and sandals on his feet. Bring the fatted calf and kill it. Let's have a feast and celebrate. For this son of mine was dead and is alive again, he was lost and is found.' So they began to celebrate." (NIV)

Although it was raining and I had drugs on me, I slowed down so I could hear the sermon that was being preached. I had heard, and even preached that sermon many times myself before I walked away from God and the church; but this time it was different. I saw myself as the prodigal who had left home, and God was the loving father who was waiting for my return.

I sat on the steps of that church, crying like a baby, and begging God to forgive me. I decided right then and there that I had to quit. Negative thoughts suddenly raced to the front of my mind, "What would be different this time? How would I succeed this time after failing so many times before? What would I have to do to increase my chances?"

When I was growing up, I had a friend named Chucky. One day, Chucky and I decided to walk down the street to the corner store. I was about 12 or 13 years old at the time. Chucky had a dog, named Champ. I hated that dog. I'm a dog lover, but I hated that one.

Chucky took Champ to the store with us. Since Champ couldn't go inside the store, Chucky handed me his leash so I could hold him until he came out. Did I tell you I hated that dog? I think Champ knew I hated him because as soon as Chucky disappeared in the store, Champ turned to me, looked me dead in my eyes and started growling. I knew I was in trouble.

Before I knew it, Champ was chasing me down the street. I was running as fast as I could but I could not get away from that dog. While I was running, I could hear people laughing and yelling something at me but I was running so fast, I couldn't hear anything they were saying. I was too busy, trying to get away from that crazy dog.

Finally, I heard someone yelling, "Let go of the leash. Let go of the leash." It hadn't dawned on me that while I was trying to get away from champ, I was still holding on to his leash. When I finally dropped the leash, Champ stopped chasing me. He ran back to the store where Chucky was.

We could get rid of a lot of our problems if we would just let go of the leash. You might have some friends that don't mean you any good. They are causing all kind of problems in your life. You need to let go of the leash. Leave them alone.

You might be in a relationship with someone who doesn't share the same goals, ambitions and values that you have. They are constantly trying to come between you and your family. You know what you have to do. Let go of the leash. Walk away from them.

You may have gotten into drugs because you were curious or wanted to fit in with the crowd. You want to quit but all of your friends are part of the drug scene. In this scenario, you need to listen to the voice of God. He is telling you loud and clear to let go of the leash.

I had to make some drastic changes in my life. Asking God to deliver me from drugs was one thing but there were some things that I had to do for myself:

1) **Stop hanging out with my old crowd.** How could I expect to stop using drugs if I was constantly surrounding myself with other junkies and dealers?

2) **Surround myself with positive people.** Positive people are those who are trying to make something of themselves -- Not the players, hustlers and cons that I used to hang out with. The problem was, I didn't know any. At least not any that wanted to have anything to do with me. So, I decided to leave Chicago and moved to St. Louis. I knew a lot of people that were in the drug game there, but I stayed away from them. It wasn't easy, but I was determined to make it this time.

3) **Never give up.** I kept getting penny-ante jobs but every time they found out about my background or criminal record, I was fired. Still, I refused to give up! I kept getting other jobs until finally I found one that didn't care about my past. With the help of my mother and some of my other relatives, I was able to make it.

4) **Have faith in yourself and God.** Although the love and support of family and friends were a vital part of my success, it was my faith in God that brought me through. Don't get me wrong, it was a tough journey and I slipped a few times along the way, but I was determined.

5) **Get up.** As I have heard people say in support group meetings, I was sick and tired of being sick and tired. As I stated earlier, just because you slip and fall in the dirt, you don't have to lay there and wallow in it. Get up. Dust yourself off and keep on stepping. If you fall down again, get up again. If you fall down again, get up again. If you keep falling down, keep getting up!

Some of our churches look at addiction as a sin. Although people sin because of their addiction, addiction itself is not a sin. It is a sickness.

One day, Oprah did a show called, "Why don't they quit?" It was a very interesting and informative look at drug addiction and the inability of addicts to kick their habits. Part of the program was very technical, dealing with different parts of the brain and how it functions. I never knew that the brain was so complex. I must've been absent the day they taught that in school.

That discussion, however, convinced a lot of people

that quitting isn't all that easy. What we must realize is that addiction is not limited to just the drug culture. It is amazing to me how many people have smoked cigarettes for years, knowing the damage that they are doing to their bodies. As hard as they have tried, they are unable to stop. A lot of them knew what the dangers were before they started. These same people, look at the person who is struggling with a drug habit and say, "Why don't you quit?"

They might argue that in our culture, cigarettes are legal and socially acceptable. My answer to that is, "so is alcohol and gambling." Look how that has devastated the lives of so many people. I would like to point out that in some cultures and sub-cultures, drug use is socially acceptable.

My father always told me that there are three steps to doing anything. He said if you follow those simple steps, there is nothing that you cannot do. With the help of the Lord, I used those steps to overcome my years of addiction. I don't claim to be an expert when it comes to recovery. There are people who have studied this area extensively and are far more qualified than I am to talk about the subject. However, this is what helped me. I believe that people will have a better chance of overcoming many of their addictions if they fully commit themselves to these three steps.

Step one: _Want to do it._

Unfortunately, this is the most difficult step of them all. When you have conquered this step, you are halfway there. Most people don't want to stop using their drug of choice because they are still enjoying it. Their friends are getting high. They cannot imagine how life would be without it. Drugs have become such an important part of who they are, they cannot see themselves going through life sober.

I say that because I didn't really want to quit. I thought I did, but the truth is, I was just tired of the consequences of my addiction. I was tired of going to jail. Besides that, I was hurting all the people that loved me. I had betrayed them so many times and in so many ways, they no longer trusted me. I was not welcome in many of their homes or even in some of their churches. As far as they were concerned, I was a leper. An outcast. A vagabond.

After spending almost a year behind bars and attending church services regularly, I thought I had beaten the drugs. I was finally clean. Eventually, I made a vow to God and to myself that when I got out, I would never stick another needle in my arm again. However, the night before I was released, the cravings were back, stronger than ever.

Although I had gone many months without drugs while I was in prison, in the back of my mind, I wanted to get high just one more time. I had not completely surrendered my heart and soul to God. Consequently, I started shooting up again shortly after I got out. It was almost as though I had never quit using. My habit was worse than ever. It was completely out of control.

"When an unclean spirit goes out of a man, he goes through dry places, seeking rest, and finds none. Then he says, 'I will return to my house from which I came.' And when he comes, he finds it empty, swept, and put in order. Then he goes and takes with him seven other spirits more wicked than himself, and they enter and dwell there: and the last state of the man is worse than the first." (Matt 12: 43-45 (NKJV)

I had gotten to the point that I realized that if I continued living that kind of life, I would soon be dead or facing a very long prison sentence. I had to be brutally honest with myself and stop trying to run games on everyone, including God. I had to accept God's help, His way. I had to make up my mind and determine that I was ready to quit. In other words, I had to **want** to quit. Then, and only then, was I ready for step two.

Step Two: *Try to do it.*

This is a difficult step as well because it takes a lot of effort. That effort is not limited to just saying no, going to church, or attending support group meetings. It takes tenacity. It takes that same tenacity, commitment and persistence to get off drugs that it took to get a hold of your drug of choice.

I used to lay awake at night dreaming and scheming of ways to get the drugs that I needed. There was no shame in my game. I did whatever it took. As far as I was concerned, going to jail was just an occupational hazard.

That is the attitude that you must have when it comes to step two. If you are not willing to do whatever it takes to overcome your addiction, you are not really trying. You can't be ashamed to ask or even beg for help. You can't be afraid to go through the pains of withdrawal. How much pain are you going through now?

You might have to go into long term treatment. If one center cannot accept you, find one that will. Don't take "no" for an answer. This is your life. Fight for it. You might have to stay away from some of your friends or relatives. Not everyone will want to see you succeed.

When I was about eleven years old, a group named, "The Coasters" recorded a song titled, "Charlie Brown." There was a different version of the song that was going around at school. In that version, some of the words were changed and there were a lot of curse words being used.

One night when our parents weren't home, my brother, Ralph and I were singing the school version of Charlie Brown, curse words and all. We were singing so loud and having so much fun, we didn't hear our mother when she came in, but she heard us. Before we could say anything, she was standing there with an ironing cord in her hand.

She looked at us and said, "Don't stop now. Keep singing." Ralph and I started crying and saying we were sorry but my mother said, "I don't want to hear I'm sorry. I want to hear Charlie Brown. Sing Charlie Brown." While she was whipping us, she made us keep singing Charlie Brown.

After that night, I never wanted to hear Charlie Brown again. As a matter of fact, every time that song came on the radio, I changed the station. That is what you must do. Change the station. If your friends are part of the drug culture, change the station. Stay away from those friends. If the places that you visit bring on temptation, change the station. Don't go to those places. There might be something, or someone that causes you to stumble. You know what you've got to do. Change the station.

You cannot be afraid of failure. Relapse is part of

recovery. If one thing doesn't work for you, try something else. People will give up on you. The important thing is, that you don't give up on yourself. Don't stop trying. Don't stop trying. Don't stop trying.

It might take a while for you to complete the first two steps. Remember, there are no shortcuts. However long it takes, you must complete them before you proceed to the third and final step.

Step Three: _Do it_.

When you reach this step, you will find that you are free from the bondage of drugs. Now you will have to become free from the effects of your years of bondage. When the children of Israel were in slavery in Egypt, they prayed to God for deliverance. Eventually, God delivered them from their bondage. However, whenever things got a little rough, they wanted to abandon their journey to the Promised Land and go back to what they knew best. They wanted to go back to Egypt. (Exodus, chapters 14 – 17)

When things get rough, times get tough and disappointment comes your way, how are you going to deal with it? Will you return to the bondage of Egypt and medicate yourself with your drug of choice, or will you march on to the Promised Land? The time will come when you will say to yourself, "What's the use?" You might even think that you can get high just one more time. That is when you will have to remember that your sobriety is not a sprint. It is a marathon.

Whatever it takes for you to remain drug free, do it. If you have to leave your family, do it. If you have to leave your friends, do it. If you have to move to another state, do it. Whatever you have to do, do it! Your life depends on it. So, do it.

Burton Barr Jr.

Lost Sheep

As I stated earlier, I am not an "expert" in this subject. My degrees are not in chemical dependency or recovery. I'm just telling you what worked for me. I'm simply one man who was strung out on every drug that you can imagine, overdosed a couple times and, by the grace of God, climbed my way from rock bottom to sobriety and a life filled with joy and purpose.

In the 15th chapter of the book of Luke, Jesus told the story of the lost sheep. The question we need to ask is, "How did that sheep end up getting lost?" I believe he nibbled himself away. There might be a herd of sheep that are just walking along, following their shepherd and the rest the sheep. At the same time, some of them will be nibbling at the grass. They will nibble a little and then look up to make sure they're still following the shepherd and the rest of the sheep. Sometimes there is that one sheep that gets so engrossed or so caught up in his nibbling that he does not look up. He's just wandering along with his head down, enjoying the grass so much that he just nibbles, and nibbles, and nibbles. When he finally does look up, he doesn't see his shepherd anywhere and he doesn't see the rest of the sheep.

He is lost. He has wondered off in the wrong direction, and he cannot find his way back. He didn't mean to get lost. He just nibbled himself away from the fold.

Our jails and prisons are full of men and women, who have nibbled themselves away from God. They have nibbled themselves away from the church. They have nibbled themselves away from everything they had ever been taught. They are not bad people. They were just nibbling.

Some of them started looking at the players that were hanging out on the street corners, smiling, styling and profiling. They became so fascinated with their fancy cars, their designer clothes and their bling, that they lost sight of their dreams, their goals and their ambitions. So they started nibbling.

Some of them were doing okay until they got curious and started nibbling on marijuana. Some of them were doing alright until they started hanging with the wrong crowds and they started nibbling with the gangs. Some of them had even gone off to college and they were doing great, until they started nibbling on alcohol. Some of them had good jobs and were respectable citizens until they started nibbling on crack. They just nibbled and nibbled until one day, they looked up and they were lost.

People start nibbling at different stages of their

life. Some start when they are young, others start when they are older. Unfortunately, some of them start nibbling while they are still in church. That's what I did. I started nibbling because I wanted to be one of the players and have some "Street Cred." I started nibbling when I started hanging out with some of the people that I worked with. Sometimes, they would get together and drink beer after work. Eventually, I started drinking with them. One Friday, they asked me to go the club with them. I still remember that night.

We were in a car on our way to a club that was located on the south side of Chicago called, "The Bird Cage" when one of them lit a joint. I had never smoked marijuana before but I didn't want them to know that I was not as cool as they thought I was. So when they passed me the joint, I took it.

I was going to church less and less. Eventually, I stopped going to church and started hanging with the players that were on the corner. I just got drunk, smoked weed, and partied all the time.

Just like that lost sheep, I had my head down and I was nibbling, and nibbling, and nibbling. And by the time I looked up, I had nibbled myself completely out of the church and into a drug habit, and then into prison.

There was a movie that came out in 1972 called "Superfly". It was the story about a big time drug dealer.

That movie messed a lot of our young men up because all they could see was a cool, well dressed player, driving around in a big, fancy car, with a fine woman and a lot of money. It glamorized the use and selling of cocaine.

Curtis Mayfield wrote the soundtrack for the movie. On any given night, all you could hear blaring from many of the nightclubs and car stereos was Superfly's song. That was the song that was playing at the end of the movie when Superfly was riding off into the sunset in his Cadillac Eldorado with his woman at his side and a briefcase full of money in the trunk. Almost every young, black man in America wanted to be like Superfly but there was another character in the movie that very few people remember. His name was Eddie.

Eddie was Superfly's crime partner but nobody wanted to be like Eddie because he didn't go riding off into the sunset at the end of the movie. As a matter of fact, the last time we saw Eddie, he was trying to make a deal with the police so he could get out of the trouble that he had gotten into.

There was a song about Eddie too, but Eddie's song wasn't as glamorous or as popular as Superfly's song. I never heard Eddie's song when I was hanging out on the street corners. They didn't play Eddie's song in the nightclubs when my boys and I were high-rolling.

About a year or so later, when I was sitting in a

prison cell, the prison disc jockey played Eddie's song on the radio one night. The name of the song was, "Eddie, You Should Know Better." That song echoed the words of many of the parents, grandparents, uncles and aunts who prayed all day and night, begging God to help us one day change our lives before it was too late.

I want to tell you about a day that I never will forget. I have told this story many times because it is a part of who I am.

It was a cold, Sunday evening in December in 1984. My body was aching because it desperately craved the drugs that it needed. I had to get some money to buy some heroin and cocaine. So I walked down 115th Street in Chicago, looking for a victim. I really didn't care who it was.

As I walked along, glancing into windows, I saw people sitting in their homes, laughing and talking and enjoying themselves with their families and their friends. I could tell that some of them had just gotten home from church. All of a sudden, my mind went back to the years before I had gotten strung out on drugs. I thought about all of the fun that I use to have with my family and my friends at Rose of Sharon Missionary Baptist Church. I could see myself sitting on the front pew with my grandmother and my little brother, listening as my pastor preached about Jesus raising Lazarus from the dead. I could see myself standing in the baptismal pool at age nine, staring into Rev. Murphy's face as he was about to baptize me and thinking to myself that one day, I was going to be like him.

I could just feel the pride that I had as I stood at my post as a junior usher. I could remember the feeling that I had years later, when at age 17, I stood in the pulpit of the Galatians Missionary Baptist Church and preached my trial sermon about Daniel in the lion's den. I thought about all of the good jobs that I'd had and how people in my church and in my community had looked up to me. Tears started rolling down my face when I remembered how proud my parents had been of me -- but all of that was over.

I was no longer that up and coming businessman in the retail industry. I was no longer that young dynamic preacher that everybody was talking about. Now I was that junkie who would con his own mother out of her last dollar so I could fill my veins with the poison that I needed.

How did I let myself get to this point? How had I messed my life up so badly? All I wanted was to be a player and make my mark in the game of the streets; but when I played the game, I lost.

When I walked down that lonely street that night, I saw something that really scared me. I saw myself. I started crying and wishing I had never left the church but it was too late. I had messed up too badly. I had nibbled myself completely away from God and into a world of hopelessness. I hated myself. I hated my life. I hated what I had become but what I hated most of all, was the hopelessness I felt. That is why I will never forget the night that I walked down 115th Street.

Burton Barr Jr.

King Heroin

---†---

In 1972, James Brown wrote and recorded a song titled, King Heroin. In it, he describes a dream that he had about a speech from a figure who turned out to be Heroin. Heroin talks about how powerful he is by making school children forget about school and attractive men and women stop caring about their appearance. He bragged about turning men into hustlers and killers and women into prostitutes and thieves.

He let the men and women who are in jail or prison know he will be waiting for them at the gate when they are released. Although he described the pain and discomfort of withdrawal, he mocked them and let them know they will pick him up again. He ended his conversation with the warning, "The white horse of heroin will ride you to Hell."

When my grandparents migrated from the south, my father's side of the family went to Chicago. My mother's side went to St. Louis. My parents separated a year or so after I was born. My mother took Ralph and moved to St. Louis. My sister already lived there with my grandparents. My father remained in Chicago with his side of the family and me. We lived in a two-story flat. We lived on the first floor along with my grandparents and Uncle Bill, my father's brother.

Dad worked in a steel foundry somewhere in K-Town. He worked very hard, trying to support my grandparents and myself but no matter how tired he was, he made Mondays our day. Those days were very special to me. We would walk around the corner to the neighborhood theater named, "The Gold." In those days, there were no malls or multiplex movie theaters.

I was around five or six years old at the time so I don't remember many of the movies that we saw. There were two movies that I will never forget: The first one was, "The Man With the Golden Arm." It starred Frank Sinatra who played the part of a heroin addict who struggled to overcome his habit. The other movie was, "Monkey On My Back." It was about a former boxer and World War II veteran who became addicted to morphine and heroin after he returned from the war. I didn't know why my father thought it was important that I saw those movies or why he talked to me about them afterwards. Whatever the reason, I decided that I would never get involved with heroin.

That was the mindset that I had years later when I started smoking marijuana. I told myself, "At least it's not heroin." When I was taking acid, I told myself, "At lease it's not heroin." When I started snorting and then shooting Duji, I told myself, "At lease it's not heroin."

That is why I will never forget the Saturday morning that Willie came to my apartment. He said, "Come on, Bub. Let's go shoot some dope." Maybe it was the way that he said it that made me uncomfortable. "Let's go shoot some dope." I didn't mess with dope. Dope was hard drugs. All I did was smoke a little reefer, pop a few pills and shoot a little Duji -- but he was talking about shooting some dope.

I asked him what kind of dope he was talking about shooting. He said, "We're going to shoot some heroin." When he said that, I felt like I was sitting in the Gold Theater again with my father, watching "*The Man With the Golden Arm*" and "*Monkey On My Back.*"

Willie and I had been shooting Duji together for weeks, along with a few other friends. So, when I told him that I didn't shoot heroin, he gave me a weird look. He said, "You don't shoot heroin?" When I said "no", he said, "Then, what do you shoot?" I said, "I don't shoot nothing but Duji." Then he said, "What do you think Duji is, fool?

People start using heroin for different reasons. For some, it might be peer pressure. For others, it could be a curiosity or a thrill of trying something new. Some might be trying to impress someone while others might try it because of a boyfriend or girlfriend. Some started because their pain medication prescription expired but were just trying to dull the pain of trying to survive in a world of hopelessness.

We see it everywhere. Hopelessness. We see it in our homes. We see it in our schools. We see it on our jobs, in our streets and in our communities. We see it in the faces of the children who don't have enough food to eat, and in the attitudes of our young people who are part of a school system that doesn't care if they receive an education or not.

We see it in the tears of that mother who is struggling and doing the best she can to raise her children by herself and we see it in the heartache of that grandmother who must raise her grandchildren because their mother is strung out on drugs.

It doesn't matter why someone started using heroin. The fact is, no one started because they wanted to be a junkie. They might know or know of someone who is strung out but some of us have an, "I can handle it" mentality.

I can shoot dope without getting strung out, because I can handle it. I can drink all the whiskey that I want without becoming an alcoholic, because I can handle it. I can do whatever I want and not worry about consequences, because I can handle it.

When I was about eleven or twelve years old, there

was a neighborhood swimming pool that was a few blocks away from my house. One day during summer vacation from school, some of my friends decided to go swimming. When I said I didn't want to go, they started teasing me, saying I couldn't swim. After a while, I agreed to go so I could show them that I could swim. The problem was, I couldn't swim. Still can't.

I remember that long walk to that building on Fillmore Avenue where the swimming pool was. My friends were talking about jumping off the diving board and other things they were going to do. I was trying to figure out how I was going get out of the mess that I had gotten myself into without drowning. I couldn't admit I couldn't swim. I couldn't punk out. But who knows? Maybe I could swim. I had never tried before.

The closer we got to the building, the more nervous I was. Soon enough, we were there. My legs felt like Jell-O as we walked up the stairs. One of the guys pulled the door handle. Nothing happened. He pulled it again. Still nothing. When we went to the other door, we saw the sign, "**CLOSED.**"

All the guys started showing their disappointment and frustration about the pool being closed, and I joined right in with them. I put on an act that was worthy of an academy award but inside, I was jumping for joy.

You might be surprised how many people's first

experience with heroin was like my swimming pool experience. They may have been hanging out or partying with some friends or acquaintances when someone offered them some. Not wanting the others know they were not cool, they tried it.

Just like I had ignored the danger and the possibility of dying from drowning, they ignored the danger of possible addiction and a life of misery and pain.

In "The Hoodlum Preacher", I told the story about the day that I was driving down a street named Davison in Detroit. Since I was just learning how to drive (actually, I was trying to teach myself), I tried to stay on safe, familiar streets. I had never driven on Davison before, but it seemed to be nice and peaceful.

I was just driving along, enjoying the sights, until all of a sudden, the sights changed. I was completely surrounded by a lot of cars and they were going fast. Real fast! What I didn't know was, at some point, with no warning at all, nice, peaceful Davison Avenue became the Davison Freeway and the entrance was the fast lane. Although it is a relatively short freeway, it seemed like it was fifty miles to me. Cars were moving so fast I couldn't get off.

When people start using heroin, they like it because they enjoy the high. It relaxes them and puts them in a mellow mood. As they continue using, with no warning at all, they went from nice, relaxing Davison Avenue, to the fast lane of the Davison Freeway and they can't get off.

They no longer use heroin to get high. It is no longer that nice, mellow recreational drug that they use to relax, chill out and nod on. Now they use it to keep from getting sick. The worst kind of sick there is, is dope sick.

People don't want to go through withdrawal. My friend, Ronald Cohen, always says that people use drugs for two reasons; to feel good, or not to feel. The drug camouflages the pain that they are feeling. So, when they are using, they are not feeling, but when they stop using, they start feeling again. If they don't know how to deal with their feelings, they will start using again.

We like to blame others for our mistakes and shortcomings. We do that because we don't want to take a hard look at ourselves. As I stated earlier, people start using drugs for different reasons, but I believe there is an underlying reason that many of us started. Notice, I said "us." I said, "us" because I don't want to try to distance myself from others who choose that life. It would be easy for me and others who were blessed to overcome our addictions, to look down our noses at the ones who are still strung out.

There are just some things I don't ever want to forget. I don't ever want to forget the night that I was crawling around in that dark ally, in a pile of dirt trying to find the needle that I had thrown away. I don't ever want to forget the night that I staged a break-in at our home and stole the money that my first wife had put away to buy food for our children. I don't ever want to forget the night that I found Linko's stash. He was the local dealer. Some of his drugs had been stolen from some of his hiding places. He put the word out that he was going to put some poison in some drugs before he hid them. I knew the drugs that I had found could have been poisoned and I could die, but I shot them anyway. I don't ever want to forget the night that I walked down 115th Street.

There are a lot of things that people are addicted to but the most common addiction that people are aware of is drugs. Professionals in the field of recovery call it chemical dependency. Some people are susceptible to addiction or have a genetic predisposition to addiction.

There are six positions about chemical dependency that many counselors in that field subscribe to. I will list four of them now and talk about the other two later.

Chemical dependency is primary, meaning *their addiction is not caused by some other thing like mental illness, moral failings or weak character.* I think people become addicted because of bad choices. Notice, I did not say that they are bad people; they just made some bad choices. Although some people have addictive personalities, they would not have gotten caught up in that lifestyle had they not chosen to experiment in that behavior.

Chemical dependency is chronic. It does not heal or subside on its own like a cold or the flu. Chronic dependency is more similar to diabetes or heart disease; it can be treated but never cured.

Although people with a chemical dependency cannot be cured, I believe they can be delivered. There are several variations of 12-Step programs and some of them are very successful. Addicts attend the meetings for different reasons. Some are ordered by a judge to attend, while others are trying to avoid jail or prison sentences. Some are trying to get out of trouble with their family members or employers while others are serious and really want help.

People often ask me how I got off drugs after being addicted for so long. Simply put, God delivered me. John 8: 36 says, "If the Son therefore shall make you free, ye shall be free indeed." Jesus asked the man at the Pool of Bethesda, *"Do you want to be made well?"* (John 5:6) Don't get me wrong, I am not against recovery programs. I attend several support group meetings and oversee one myself.

Chemical Dependency is progressive. It *gets worse over time. If not treated, it eventually damages the body, mind and spirit.*

In 1969, when I started snorting and then, shooting heroin. I went from spending $3 on weekends to spending $20 every day. Eventually, my addiction to heroin and cocaine was costing an average of, $200-500 per day. Although it has been almost 30 years since I have used drugs, the damage that it did to my body is still evident.

Choices have consequences. Just because you have been delivered from something does not mean that you will not have to face the consequences of those choices.

Chemical dependency is fatal and it may cause death if left unchecked. Vital organs of the body may become too damaged to function. Chemical dependency deaths take on one of three forms: overdose, accident or suicide. However, treatment combined with the ongoing work of recovery can result in recovering addicts having full and healthy lives.

This might sound crazy, but addicts often want drugs that caused other addicts to overdose and die. That way, they knew the drugs that they were buying were really good. We thought we were smarter than the people that died. I knew a lot of people who fell into that category. I was one of them.

Addictions are not only formed because of family history, but some people become addicted to certain substances because of their associations. People want to be liked, therefore, some of them try things that their friends are doing. Sometimes they are just trying to impress someone of the opposite sex. The problem is, they might have a genetic predisposition to addiction but their friend does not.

My friends, opioid use in the United States are completely out of control. We house more than 22% of the world's prisoners. Most of the crimes that the inmates committed were drug related, meaning, they were either caught with drugs, they committed a crime to get drugs or they were high when they committed a crime.

The number of drug users are steadily increasing. In 2016, there were more than 200,000 new heroin users. There were 63,600 drug overdoses that year and opioids were the cause of 4,229 of them. The death toll keeps rising. Every day, approximately 142 Americans die from drug overdoses. That's more than 70,000 Americans that die every year.

What those statistics don't show is the collateral damages. Thousands of people are murdered every year in this country over drug wars and turf battles. Innocent people are being robbed and killed by addicts who need a fix, or the addict, himself, is killed because he trusted the wrong person.

In drug culture, when new dealers come into a neighborhood, they often give away sample bags of heroin to potential customers so they can steal them away from their regular dealers. Sometimes, the established dealers do giveaways when they get a new product. They use the addicts as guinea pigs.

The way some dealers do the "giveaways" is very demeaning. They would spread the word that they will give out some free samples at a certain time. When the time came, they would throw a few handfuls of bags of heroin on the ground into a crowd of addicts. That is what happened to my friend, Fuzzy.

When I was about 14 years old, Gip and some other friends of mine introduced me to a new kid that had just moved into the neighborhood. His name was, Fuzzy. When they told me his name, I started teasing him. I said Fuzzy Wuzzy was a bear. Fuzzy Wuzzy lost his hair. Then Fuzzy Wuzzy wasn't Fuzzy, Wuzzy?

He started chasing me down the street. By the time he caught up with me, we were both laughing. From that time on, we became the best of friends.

Fuzzy lived on Roosevelt Road and Christiana Avenue above a tavern that was named, "The Heat Wave." He lived there with his father, grandmother and his brother, Billy. He was about a year older than me and very streetwise. His grandmother used their apartment as a gambling establishment and she also sold bootleg liquor after hours.

I was kind of jealous of Fuzzy and the way he lived. He didn't have a curfew and he had complete freedom to come and go as he pleased and to do whatever he wanted. He didn't go to school and he always had plenty of money and was a sharp dresser. He was like "Fonzie" on Happy Days.

We had been through a lot together during our teenage years. We played together, fought together, and almost died together. Yeah, Fuzzy was one of my best friends.

When I started snorting and shooting heroin, I convinced some of my friends to do the same and Fuzzy was one of them. As a matter of fact, I was the one who first stuck a needle in his arm. We got high together quite often.

Years later, I moved to St. Louis, Missouri. One day I received a phone call from my mother telling me that Fuzzy was dead. What bothered me more was when Ralph told me the way that he had died. Fuzzy got one of those free giveaway samples of heroin one day, but it was laced with arsenic. His grandmother found him lying on the floor in his bedroom with the needle still in his arm. That was the same room where he and I shot up many times.

Almost everyone who shot or snorted some of it died. I guess that was their way of getting rid of some junkies. Fuzzy was one of them but he was not the only friend or acquaintance of mine whose death was drug related.

The Queen

In the drug culture, heroin is known as boy and cocaine is called girl. If heroin is the king of drugs, cocaine is certainly the queen. It doesn't matter whether you snort it, smoke it or shoot it, the risk of becoming addicted is the same.

When I decided it was time to quit shooting heroin, I was afraid that I would go through withdrawal. I didn't want to do that. As I stated earlier, the worst kind of sick there is, is dope sick. When I was talking to another junkie about my dilemma, he said, "The best way to cleanse the heroin from your system is to shoot some cocaine." It made perfect sense to me, since heroin and cocaine were opposites.

So, when I got off work one evening, I copped a quarter bag of cocaine. I went home and dumped the whole bag into the cooker, put some water in it, and drew it up in the syringe. I went into the bathroom, found my favorite vein and ran it.

It seems like I heard a bell ring in my head. There was a feeling that came over me like I had never felt before. I got scared. My heart was rushing. My mind was rushing. My eyes were rushing. What had I found here? While the needle was still hanging from my arm, I stuck my hand in my pocket to see how much money I had left. I had to get some more of that!

I thank God the cocaine that I had purchased was not as potent as it should have been. Running a quarter bag like I did should have killed me. While I was walking back to the spot to get another bag, I knew I had finally met my match. Heroin couldn't do it. Reefer couldn't do it. Alcohol couldn't do it, however, after shooting cocaine the very first time, I knew, without a doubt, that I was whipped. I was hooked, big time. I had found the "girl" that would completely control my life for years.

Shooting cocaine is nothing like shooting heroin. You might shoot heroin several times a day but if it is any good, you will never shoot it back to back. You will nod off for a while or "get your sick off", and then get some more a few hours later. With cocaine, as soon as you finish shooting or smoking it, you want more. Sometimes people will shoot or smoke cocaine for days at a time.

Cocaine became popular in some communities in the 70s after the movie, "Superfly" came out. Everybody wanted to be like Priest, the flamboyant, successful dealer. In those days, cocaine was an acceptable drug. They called it, "The rich man's high." It gained that distinction because of its clientele, but the price might have had a little to do with it. You could get a bag of weed for $5.00 or a bag of heroin for $10.00. The cost of a bag of cocaine was $25.00.

People carried small vials filled with cocaine with them and wore small coke spoons on chains around their necks. It was used while sitting at tables in night clubs or in other public areas but some people, including me, were uncomfortable spending that much money so most of us stuck to lesser priced drugs like weed, pills and boy.

There was a major incident in the 1980 drug world that that made more people want to try it. Comedian, Richard Pryor was badly burned while freebasing. Freebasing is purifying cocaine by mixing it with baking soda and water and cooking it in test tubes. Most people had never heard of it until Richard Pryor almost killed himself.

After that incident, more people wanted to try basing. They figured, if that is what people like Richard Pryor do to get high, it must be cool. This is the mentality of the average drug user; if someone overdosed from a batch of drugs, everybody wanted some of that. They thought it had to be some good stuff. The 1980s introduced many communities to a new, powerful, life changing drug called crack. It is highly addictive and very cheap.

I started shooting cocaine in 1984. I had a good job working as a salesperson at JC Penny in a Chicago suburb.

Although most of the dealers sold $25.00 bags, called quarter bags. Some started selling dime bags. That made the drug more affordable and was good for people who just wanted a small amount.

I started by speed balling. That is mixing heroin and cocaine together and shooting or snorting it. When mixed together, the cocaine stimulates the users and the heroin mellows them out. It gives the user the best of both worlds. The heroin satisfies the addicts need for opioids while the cocaine arouses them. The problem is, cocaine makes the user keep going back for more. That is the nature of the beast.

Cocaine is conning and deceiving. It lures you in, using an appeal that is almost seductive. Most people don't realize they are addicted. They think they can quit any time they want. They just don't want to quit because they like it.

I was talking to my cellie one day when I was in prison. For those of you who are not familiar with the term, that means cellmate. I was telling him about some of my experiences and things that I had gone through since I started using cocaine. He said I sounded like I was talking about a woman. After thinking about it, he was right. My addiction to cocaine was like being in a love/hate relationship with a woman. I didn't want her but I couldn't live without her. She was good to me but she wasn't good for me.

In one of my earlier books, I talked about the time I was visiting the home of my friends, Vernon and Zetta one Thanksgiving. Vernon loved "dusties" (old records) and he had a large collection of them. He played a record by The Stylistics named, "Children of the Night."

While the record was playing, I sat back on the couch with my eyes closed. Although I had heard that song many times before, it was as if I was hearing the words for the very first time. I could visualize myself, years earlier, when I was strung out and living in a world of hopelessness. There were so many nights that the empty, restless feeling took control of me. I couldn't fight it, so I walked the streets in search of the girl.

Although the Stylistics weren't talking about drugs in the song, that was how I felt. I had become one of the children of the night who was constantly in search of the company that I craved so badly. Cocaine. Nothing or no one was more important, not even family, friends, children or jobs; everything came second to the queen, Miss Caine. I walked the streets, sometimes all night long, longing for her company.

I was on a mission. A popular phrase that was being used at the time was, "Chasin Jasin" (Chasing Jason). That is when someone is desperately searching for drugs or money to get them. Every addict is chasing something. The problem is, most of us don't know what it is.

When I was in prison, I had a recurring dream. I had a syringe filled with heroin or cocaine. I wrapped my belt around my arm and found my favorite vein. Just as I was about to stick the needle in my arm, I woke up. That is what the chase is like. Looking back, I think addicts don't know it, but what they are really chasing is death. Unfortunately, too many of them are catching him.

During the last few years of my addiction, I was at my worst. I was no longer the slick talking con man who could convince people to trust me with their money or valuables. Instead, I was a junkie who would steal anything from anyone. When my uncle died, my aunt asked me to move in with her. That was a huge mistake. I robbed her blind. She got so upset with me, she pulled a gun on me one day. I thought she was going to shoot me. The next day, I stole her gun.

Addicts choose drugs over family and friends by the choices they make. It may not be intentional. Let's say, you are supposed to be someplace at a certain time for something important. You decide to take a hit before you leave. Then another. Then another. Then another. You never make it to your appointment. If you do, you're so late that it doesn't matter.

A friend of mine's mother passed away. She got to the funeral in plenty of time, but she decided to sit in a car with her sister and smoke some crack before the service started. By the time they finished, the service was almost over. In the words of Chaka Khan, "Once you get started, it's hard to stop."

The reality is, I think what I wanted to escape from was the dreams that I had shattered. I had been a young, sought after preacher but I walked away from the church. I was a respected businessman in the retail industry, but I lost control of my drinking. I was moving up the political ladder, working for one of the first black US Congressmen, but I was nodding off in meetings, because I was high. I was a Sergeant in the Marines, but I was kicked out and sent to prison because of my addictions.

I had thrown all of those dreams away. My life was over. My dreams were shattered. All I could do was think about what I used to be or what I could have been. Like millions of addicts, I was living in a world of hopelessness. That was the reality that I and so many others are trying to escape. That is what I mean when I say we don't want to feel.

There are a lot of things that might cause someone to stumble; the death of a loved one, the loss of a job or the breakup with a spouse or significant other. It is easy to lose your focus when you are hurting. As the saying goes, "hurt people, hurt people." What they don't tell you is that hurt people also hurt themselves.

Several people confronted or tried to help me with my drug problem, but no one tried harder than my cousin Rosemary. She was more like a sister than a cousin and was actually the reason I finally went to treatment. Although I loved her, I wanted her to leave me alone and mind her business.

I ran a lot of con games on people but the only ones that really bothered me were the games that I played on my family. Most of the cons were just coke lies. Addicts can easily fool their loved ones because they love them and want to believe them. Even when the loved ones know that the addict is lying, they want to give us the benefit of the doubt. They really want to believe that this time, their loved one is telling the truth.

Sometimes God will let a parent know when his or her child is in trouble. When I was in the Marines, I was stationed in California. I had gotten into some trouble and was sent to the brig. I didn't tell my parents about it because I didn't want them to worry. I was called to the chaplain's office one day. When I got there, I found out my father was on the phone. He told me that God had told him that I was in trouble.

It is not always that drastic. Sometimes, a feeling will come over you and you just can't shake it. On October 13, 2017, my publisher's friend lost her 21 year old daughter to a cocaine overdose. Her name was Deshaye

Collins. Deshaye left the house to go to a party. Her mother begged her not to go because she had a bad feeling. She told her mother she needed to live her own life and to stop worrying about her. She kissed her mom and went to the party. Someone had laced some cocaine with something. Deshaye collapsed and died in the back of an Atlanta night club.

She was not a bad person, in fact, she was a sweet, loving young lady. She loved her mother and her little sister. She just did what hundreds of thousands of young people do every day. I was sorry to hear about his friend and her tragic loss. He asked what would I have said to Deshaye to keep her from going out that night.

To be honest, I don't know what I would have told her. There are no cookie cutter responses. What might reach one person will have no effect on another. Before I talk to anyone, I ask God for His guidance. What I might have done that night was ask Deshaye if I could pray with her before she left. Notice, I said pray with her, not for her.

Holding hands with her and her mother, I might have prayed for her safety and for God to direct her path. I believe God would have told me what else I should say. Maybe something that I would have said during the prayer would have given her pause.

Deshaye's story gave me the inspiration that I

needed to finally write this book. Imagine that was your son or daughter. It could be. We are losing our children to drug overdoses at an alarming rate. I pray for Deshaye's mother, Monica Hill, almost every night. I've lost a lot of friends and relatives to drugs, mostly cocaine. The queen can be a charming, yet cunning drug.

I'm reminded of this by a song, "The Snake", by Oscar Brown Jr. On a very cold evening, a young lady was walking through the woods on her way home. She came across a snake that was lying by the side of the road. As she came closer she could see that the snake had been injured and was nearly frozen to death.

The woman felt compassion for the snake, so she picked it up, wrapped her coat around it and took it home with her. When she got home she fed the snake, placed it in front of the fireplace and nursed it all night long. The next morning, before she left for work, she changed the bandages, set plenty of food out for the snake and made sure that the heat was left on high.

That evening, when she got home, she was surprised to see that the snake's wounds were healing and its condition was no longer critical. The snake was even crawling around on the floor, laughing and playing.

The woman was so happy that the snake was feeling better, she ran over to it, picked it up, and started hugging and kissing it. While she was hugging the snake, it hauled off and gave her a vicious bite on her neck.

The woman dropped the snake and fell back in a state of shock. She grabbed her neck and with tears in her eyes she said, "How could you do this to me after all I have done for you? You know your bite is poisonous and now I am going to die. How could you do this to me?"

The snake just looked at her and said, "Shut up, silly woman. You knew I was a snake before you took me in."

Using cocaine is the worst decision that many of us have ever made. As I stated earlier, I have lost a lot of friends and family members to cocaine. Not all of them died, but where the queen took them was almost just as bad.

I first met Linda in the early 1980s. She lived down the street from me. Boy, was she fine. She was beautiful, sexy and smart, and she knew it. Every man in that part of town wanted her, including me. I talked to her a few times. We even drank beer and smoked weed together sometimes but that was as far as I, or anyone else could get.

I saw her again in 1988. I had moved back to St. Louis after my father was killed. I left Chicago to get away from shooting heroin and cocaine but when I got to St. Louis, I started smoking crack with my cousins and their friends.

Burton Barr Jr.

I was looking to buy a ten dollar rock when I ran into Linda. She still looked good, but a little different. We talked for a while, then I told her where I was going and why. She offered to give me oral sex if I would split the rock with her. I couldn't believe it. The beautiful, sexy, intelligent woman who many of us looked at as a goddess a few years ago, was offering herself for what amounted to a five dollar rock. Crack had taken this young lady, with a promising future and put her on the streets.

Another one of my friends, Erma, had a loving husband, a beautiful home and nice family. They both had good jobs and everything to look forward to, but Erma's husband died suddenly. Shortly thereafter, she started using drugs to help her deal with her grief and was eventually introduced to the queen. Within a year, Erma had lost her job and her house.

I grew up living around the corner from one of my close friends, Red. He had always been the life of the party. Like many of us, Red got heavily involved in drugs. He met the queen in an elaborate cocaine scheme and that was his downfall as well. He was found in a hotel room with his throat cut.

I met Butch around the same time that I met Fuzzy but I didn't start off teasing him like I did Fuzzy. Butch was bigger than both of us. He was the cousin of my girlfriend, Betty Jean. He was in the marines and served in Vietnam.

Like so many others, he came back from the war with a drug habit. We used to shoot up together. Like it was with Fuzzy, I was living in St. Louis when I got word that Butch had overdosed and died.

One day after work, I also overdosed on heroin but was lucky I wasn't alone when it happened. There were a few of us in my apartment at the time. I pressed the needle into my vein and allowed the heroin take over. My legs became weak as I fell back against the wall. Slowly descending to the floor, I uttered, "This is some good ----." The next thing I remember was waking up on the couch. Someone said Poopy shot some salt in my arm to bring me out of it. I never would've thought that a guy named Poopy would be the one that God used to save my life.

I overdosed on cocaine several times. One time, my heart was beating so fast I thought I was going to die but I shot some heroin to bring me down. After I realized I wasn't going to die, I bought more cocaine. Crazy, isn't it?

I could have died during any of those episodes, not to mention the many times that I was confronted by the stick-up man after leaving a cop house. I even faced people with guns aimed at me, trying to take my dope. They either hesitated or I did something to distract them so I could get away. Every time, God allowed me to get away.

Heroin and crack have destroyed the lives of so

many people and families. Most of the men and women who are incarcerated are there for drug offences. They are not drug lords or kingpins, they are petty criminals with drug problems. They need rehab, not prison.

I had just finished preaching at a church service one Sunday at one of the state prisons in Missouri. One of the inmates that regularly attend my services came up to me. He introduced me to the young man that was with him. It was his son. I was glad he brought his son to church with him but I was a little saddened that it happened while they were both in prison.

A friend and I were shooting up in my bedroom one day. The door was closed but I didn't know it was cracked. When I looked up, I saw my 12 year old nephew, Dewayne, in the living room looking at me. He had always looked up to me. I don't know how seeing that affected him. We never talked about it.

I had always thought I was only hurting myself with the lifestyle that I was living. It wasn't until years later that I learned how my choices affected my children and many other young people around me. When I talk to the men and women in the prisons, I challenge them to be good examples for their children, nieces, nephews and other young people when they are released.

The first time that I went to rehab, I thought it was going to be easy. After all, I had always said I could quit any time I wanted to. After I checked in, I was taken to a room and assigned to a bed. Shortly after that, a nurse came in and gave me a shot. I thought the shot was going to cure me. Right.

I have to admit that sounds crazy but you have to remember, I shot up in an alley while I was on the way to rehab. So I was high when I got there.

Being successful at kicking a drug habit is like being successful at anything else. You have to work at it. When we were children, my grandparents had a piano in their home. It was more of a decoration since neither of them played. We lived in a two family flat. I lived on the second floor with my parents and my brother, Ralph. My grandparents lived on the first floor.

Ralph and I had always wanted to learn how to play the piano. All we were able to play was, "Mary had a little lamb" and "Twinkle, twinkle little star" with one finger. Eventually, we talked our parents into letting us take piano lessons. We were excited when we found out the piano teacher was coming on Saturday.

We made a list of all of the songs that we wanted to learn how to play. We wrote down the names of all of our favorite songs that we heard in church. We listened to the radio every day and added some of the songs that we liked to the list. We figured that since the piano lesson was going to last an hour, we should be able to learn how play about 10 or fifteen songs. Maybe even twenty. We were so excited, we could hardly sleep that Friday night.

When the teacher arrived, we were ready. I handed her the list of songs and sat on the stool. She didn't even look at the list. She had us play some crazy exercise over and over again for the entire hour. Then she told us to practice that exercise every day for an hour and she left.

Ralph and I were in shock. We looked at each other, trying to figure out what had just happened. I looked at the list of songs that we had prepared. I thought we would be able to play some of the songs that were on our list. I was so disappointed, I never took another piano lesson. As a result, all I am able to play today is, "Mary had a little lamb" and "Twinkle, twinkle little star" with one finger.

Nothing that is worthwhile happens overnight. To be successful at anything, it takes hard work. That includes recovering from an addiction. You have to work at it. No pain, no gain. If you are serious about your recovery, you have to give your all. Otherwise, you're just playing, "Mary had a little lamb" and "Twinkle, twinkle little star" with one finger.

Cocaine is deceitful. It makes you paranoid. It will have you seeing and hearing things that are not there. There were times when I thought someone was hiding in the closet or peeking in my window. I lived on the second floor. One day, I was so high, I thought my father was on top of a telephone pole in the alley, looking in the window. He was 78 years old.

I had just finished shooting up one night when I thought I heard something in Ralph's bedroom. He wasn't home, so I went in to take a look around. The power in our house was off because we didn't pay the electric bill. We had a drop lamp in the kitchen that ran from the building next door. The cord wasn't long enough to reach all of the way into Ralph's room, so I pulled out my cigarette lighter.

After looking around the room, I decided to look under the bed. I got down on my knees and flicked my lighter but I couldn't see all of the way under the bed. So I reached under the bed as far as I could with the lighter still burning. Since the box spring was kind of old and ragged, there were some loose strands hanging from the bottom. The flame from the lighter got too close to one of the strands and the box springs caught fire. I pulled the mattress off of it and stood it against the wall so I could put the fire on the box springs out. What I didn't know was that the mattress was burning too, and the flame caught onto the curtains.

I was able to get the fire out without any more damage. Dad came up and helped me take the mattress and box springs to the alley. When Ralph came home that night, I think he was a little surprised to see that he didn't have a bed anymore. Boy, I didn't think he could get that mad. I just thank God that I didn't burn the whole house down.

Those are the kind of really dumb things that cocaine will make people do. I have seen people search the floor, looking for a piece of a rock that they may have dropped. The crazy thing is, they are looking on the floor in a room that they were not smoking in. They were getting high in the basement but they are looking on the floor in the living room.

I sold cocaine during several periods in my life. Sometimes it was to make money, other times it was to supplement my own use. There were times when I literally ran and hid from customers so I could have more coke for myself, especially if I was running short of product. Crack wasn't out yet, so most people free-based.

My doorbell rang one day when I was getting high. When I peeped out, I saw Gip and Don standing on the porch. I knew they wanted to buy some coke so I didn't answer. Sometime later, I needed to pick up something. I went out the back door so no one would see me. While I was walking through the alley, I heard someone say, "There he is." It was Gip and Don.

I ran down the alley and ducked in a gangway. I made my way to another gangway and hid in a basement. When I thought the coast was clear, ran down the alley, climbed over my back fence and hid in the basement. I don't think I would have made dealer of the year.

Looking back on that incident, it makes me laugh, but there was nothing funny the time Little Joey came by. Joey drove a school bus for one of the companies that served the Chicago area.

I had just re-upped when Joey came by. He had dropped the students off at school, so he had a few hours before he had to pick them up and take them home. He bought some cocaine and went in the living room to cook and smoke it. I was in the back bedroom, cutting and mixing the coke. About a half hour later, I heard his little feet coming through the kitchen. He wanted to buy more coke.

I sold it to him. About a half hour later, I heard those little feet again, and again, and again. That went on for several hours until I cut him off. I told him I had run out of drugs and would have more that evening. I was concerned because it was almost time for him to pick the children up from school and take them home.

Brian Cavanaugh told a story that has great meaning. I embellished it a little but the implication is the same. A little boy was playing in his backyard one day when he noticed a huge rock that was in the middle of the yard. He decided to move the rock so he would have more room to play. He pushed the rock as hard as he could, but it would not budge. He tried pushing it from another angle but still, the rock would not move. Becoming frustrated, the boy sat down and tried to shove the stubborn rock with his feet. The rock would not move.

His father glanced out the window and saw him struggling with the gigantic rock. He went outside and watched his son as he toiled intensively, trying to move the rock. Finally, he said, "Son. Are you using all of your strength?" The boy said that he was. His father stood there, watching his son as he strained and struggled with the enormous rock. He asked his son again, "Are you using all of your strength?" Again, the boy said that he was.

His father stood there, watching his son grunting, groaning and sweating as he desperately tried to move the humongous rock. He said, "Son. Are you sure you are using all of your strength?" The boy was almost in tears when he said, "Yes Dad. I am using all of my strength." His father put his hand on his son's shoulder and said, "Son. You are not using all of your strength. I know, because you haven't asked me to help you."

Are you trying to move that giant rock called addiction by yourself? You don't have to do it alone. God is watching you. He is asking, "Are you using all of your strength?"

Dr. Feel Good

More and more people are becoming addicted to prescription drugs. Some of them were involved in an accident, had some kind of surgery, had dental work done or just had some kind of illness. Whatever the case, the pain that they were feeling may have been somewhat unbearable. They did what they were supposed to do. They took the medicines that were legally prescribed to them by their doctor, but something unexpected happened. The medication not only relieved their pain, they liked how it made them feel. It made them feel good.

Many of them had never taken any illegal drugs. They had never gotten involved with heroin, cocaine or any other street drug. They were typical working class people, but they were becoming dependent on the medicine. They were looking forward to taking it. They were getting hooked. When their medicine ran out, they called their doctor and requested a refill.

Some of them may have been former users. When they took the prescribed medicine, it awakened something within. They may have been clean for quite some time and managed to stay away from their drug of choice, but these drugs are not illegal. They were prescribed to them by a reputable doctor. Their name was on the bottle. The problem is, they are opioids. They are addictive. If used improperly, they are trouble. Now they are addicted.

When their prescription runs out, they have to get their pills from somewhere else. They can't go to Walgreens or CVS anymore. They can't go to the neighborhood pharmacy. They have to find someone else to get what they need. Enter, Dr. Feel Good.

There are some dealers who don't sell hard drugs. They just sell the ones that require prescriptions. I call them Dr. Feel Good. Most of their customers are people whose prescriptions have run out, or young people who are looking for a good time.

Some believe that marijuana is a gateway to hard drugs and for some people, this is true. However, it seems like the gateway to hard drugs for others is the abuse of prescription drugs. The drugs are not just a problem for them. Sometimes their children find them and they try them because the heard about them from their friends or they were curious. Either way, the path that they were on led them to Dr. Feel Good.

After my father was killed in 1988, I left Chicago and moved to St. Louis. One of the reasons was I wanted to get away from heroin. The other reason was I owed Linko, the neighborhood dealer, for some drugs. Since I didn't have his money, I figured it was a good time to change area codes.

When I got to St. Louis, I was glad to be away from heroin and the crowd that I hung with. I moved in with my cousin and his family. There was a corner of the basement that was almost like a private room. That was where I lived. Unfortunately, that was also where my cousin and some of her friends smoked crack. I went from shooting heroin to smoking crack.

I supported my habit by passing bad checks and running a few con games. I was arrested one night. The police officer handcuffed me, put me in his car and drove into a dark alley. I thought he was going to beat me up. Instead, he told me to get out of St. Louis and never come back. He said I'd better not even show up in court. It was time to find another city. I couldn't go back to California. I couldn't go back to Chicago. I had to leave St. Louis. I chose Detroit.

My first wife, Jeri, and I got back together. We had a nice apartment and I had a good job driving a fork lift. I stayed away from drugs and alcohol. I had gotten back in church and everything was going fine. Then I caught a very bad cold.

One of the medicines that I took was Vicks Nyquil. After taking that for a few days, I felt better, but like some people do while taking prescription drugs, I kept taking it after the cold was gone. I wasn't doing drugs. I wasn't drinking liquor. All I was doing after work was drinking my Nyquil.

I went to a drug store or convenience store on my way home and bought a bottle of Nyquil. When I got close to home, I turned the bottle up and gulped it all down. Sometimes I bought another bottle so I could take one home with me. I didn't have to worry about Jeri or anyone seeing it because it was just cough syrup. If anyone questioned me about it, I would start coughing.

I always waited until I was close to home before I drank it because I didn't want to take a chance getting pulled over. I was wanted in Missouri and I was in no shape to be driving.

I used to wonder why people called the thing above the sink in the bathroom a medicine cabinet. Most of the time, the only medicine that was in there was a bottle of aspirin. Everything else that was in there just helped make you look or smell good. That was where we kept our tooth brush, toothpaste, comb, brush, cologne, Afro King, Afro Queen, curl activator and all the other important stuff (perhaps I digressed back to the 70s and 80s).

To my surprise, some people actually keep medicine in their medicine cabinet. There is nothing wrong with that but there are some prescription medicines that

the medicine cabinet might not be the best place for them. Besides curious children and rambling teenagers, there are also guests that might get a little nosey.

One Saturday night, Chucky came to my house. He had some pills that he called, Trees (short for Christmas Trees). I took two of them and then we walked down Roosevelt Road to the club. He told me to watch myself because those trees would sneak up on me. Boy was he right. About an hour or so later, everything was just a big blur. I tried to find Chucky so we could get out of there but I kept bumping into people. Finally I decided to get out of there and go home.

It was about a five-block walk down Roosevelt from Albany to Christiana, and for five blocks I was leaning on one building after another. I don't know how I managed to get across any of those streets, but I had never been so glad to almost see my house. When I was about three houses away from my door, I saw a gang of men coming towards me. It looked like it was about 30 of them. I found out later that this "gang" consisted of only four men.

Nevertheless, when they saw the condition I was in, they robbed me, taking my wallet and my watch. I was so high, I couldn't fight, I couldn't run and I couldn't yell. All I could do was just lie there against that building while they were hitting me and going through my pockets. I was hoping they would hurry up and finish robbing me so I could go in the house and lie down.

The next day I found out that Chucky had teamed up with my friend, Gip, to look for me at the club. They said that one minute they saw me and the next minute they didn't. At that moment, I knew that I didn't want to mess with any more Trees.

Another pill that I started taking was called, Reds (short for Red Devils). I used to take them with a friend of mine named, Mike. We became friends after his brother was murdered. Mike was always trying to get me to stop shooting dope. He talked about how bad my arms looked, so he turned me on to Reds. We stayed high all of the time, drinking fifths of gin and dropping Reds.

I bought some pills called, Whites (short for White Cross). They are uppers or speed. They sure did that. They were so small and inexpensive. One day, I took more than I should have. I was up for two days.

I went to Fuzzy's one Sunday afternoon. Some of his friends were there and they were drinking and shooting some T's and Blues, the poor man's heroin. I had never heard of them before but when they asked me if I wanted some, I said yes. Fuzzy shot the drugs into my arm but it must have been too much for the first time because I overdosed and passed out. When I came to, I was lying on the kitchen floor.

Later that evening, when the drugs started wearing

off, my shoulder was really hurting. Dad went with me to Cook County Hospital where I learned my shoulder was dislocated.

There are lots of other pills that people buy from Dr. Feel Good. I just told you about the ones that I have experience with. Bottom line, addiction to prescription drugs is a serious problem.

I told you about my struggle with Vicks Nyquil. In the 60s and 70s, Robitussin cough syrup was used and abused by teenagers and others to get high. It forced drug stores to change the way they shelved it.

Robitussin wasn't the only thing that changed retail store policies. The more roadblocks the stores put in front of the drug community, the more creative drug users and dealers got. Murine had to stop putting eye droppers in the boxes with the medicine because they were being used in place of syringes to shoot heroin with. It had gotten to the point where we wouldn't buy the Murine, we just stole the eye droppers from the boxes.

McDonalds had to stop giving out those long, tiny spoons with their coffee. Dealers were using the spoons to measure heroin. They called them, "Mac Spoons." Three spoons full equaled a dime bag.

During my research for this book, I read some books and talked to a few people on the subject of addiction and recovery. My friend, Ronald Cohen was very helpful. He is a recovery specialist, but most of what is covered in this book is from experience. It is the same as when I minister to the men and women in the jails and prisons. I let them know that what I tell them is not from a book (excluding excerpts from the Bible). I want them to know that I have been through what many of them are going through.

People are hurting. That is why many of them started using drugs. Some of them may have started with prescription pills. Others may have started with alcohol or marijuana. We cannot judge them because we don't know the circumstances that led to their addiction.

Happy Hour

I came from a family of alcoholics. One of my earliest memories was sitting on a barstool next to my grandfather in a tavern named, Jack's Foxhole. I was five or six years old. He picked me up from school every day and we would walk to the tavern on our way home. I would drink a glass of milk and he drank something else. That was our daily routine.

My father, most of my uncles, cousins and even some of my aunts had drinking problems. Some were more serious than others. Dad quit drinking after he accepted his call to the ministry. At first, he was a closet drinker. Ralph would find his stash and give them to my mother. He finally quit altogether.

The most noticeable and remembered alcoholic in my family was my Uncle Hebert. He was the neighborhood drunk. Do you remember Otis Campbell on the Andy Griffith show? Uncle Hebert was a nice, likeable, hardworking gentleman, but on the weekends, he was an entirely different person.

I still remember him staggering down Christiana on Friday evenings after he got off from work. I think he stopped at Jack's Foxhole while on his way home. Sometimes, Aunt Ruth would help him get down the street and up the stairs. She was so embarrassed.

Ralph and I used to watch the wrestling matches on TV every Friday night with our parents. We were huge wrestling fans. One day, Uncle Herbert came to our house to visit for a while. Somehow, the subject of wrestling came up. He said he was going to take Ralph and me to the wrestling match that Friday night. We were so excited.

Friday night came, but Uncle Hebert didn't. As excited as we were earlier that week, we were five times more disappointed that night. I guess he just couldn't get past Jack's Foxhole.

My parents explained that sometimes, Uncle Hebert has the best intentions. He might have meant it when he said it, but it was the liquor talking or he started drinking and forgot. Either way, it hurt just as bad. It must have; I still remember it 60 years later.

People say or promise things when they have been drinking. We all do. We meant what we said, when we said it. It sounded good and even made sense, but when we got sober the next day, we regret saying what we said, if we can remember it.

Some of the things that we say might be promises or ideas that we have, while others might be us simply telling someone off. In some cases, we are letting someone know how we really feel; we are getting stuff off our chests. These may be things that we had been holding in for some time.

Sometimes we make promises to our spouses or significant others. We promise to take them someplace or give them something. We must be careful when it comes to making promises, especially to children because some things might affect them for years, if not for life. They don't know that it was the alcohol talking.

When we were teenagers, my friends and I formed a social club called, "The Mack Men." We were not a gang. We were just a group of guys from the neighborhood that partied, played ball and hung out together.

There was a group of guys from another neighborhood that would sometimes try to crash the parties and start trouble. They were part of Fat Nash's gang. One night some of them came in and wanted to fight, so we all went outside.

Butch was bigger than the rest of us and the only one with any gang fighting experience so he stepped forward and challenged Saul, who was their captain and Fat Nash's right hand. Saul said he wasn't going to waste his time fighting a chump like Butch so he called one of his boys, Clint, to do the fighting. So Butch said he was not going to fight a chump like Clint. So he told Clint to pick someone in our group that he wanted to fight. Clint picked me.

Clint was a big, country boy. He was almost a foot taller than I was and he outweighed me by almost thirty pounds. I didn't care; I thought I was Muhammad Ali. Besides that, the beer and whiskey that I had been drinking at the party gave me all of the confidence that I needed.

I started dancing around and throwing jabs like I had seen Ali do on TV. I kept dancing in and jabbing him and then dancing back before he could hit me. Clint was too big to keep up with me. I was Ali and he was Sonny Liston. Everyone was cheering me on and saying, "Go Bub, go!" Then, the whiskey started talking to me. It said, "Grab him and body slam him." So I moved in and grabbed Clint around his waist and tried to pick him up.

When I woke up---I was in my bathroom lying on the floor and someone was putting wet towels and cold water on my face. I asked somebody what had happened. They kept asking me why I grabbed Clint. The whiskey told me to do it.

We live in a society where drinking alcohol is glamorized. In the movies, when someone gets home from work, the first thing that he or she does is pour themselves a drink. All of the cool, successful people drank.

A common phrase and time in America is called, "Happy Hour." That coincides with the time when many people get off work. Bars offer discounted drinks to customers during that time, but happy hour is not just an hour. In some cases, it lasts two or even three hours.

Some people use that as an opportunity to avoid rush hour. So they sit in a bar, drinking with friends and co-workers for a few hours, then they get in their cars and drive home. I loved it.

I was one of those people who thought I could drive better after having a few drinks. I remember the years when I stopped at Walgreens every day after work. That was when they sold liquor. I was there so often, the clerk at the liquor counter didn't ask what I wanted. When he saw me walk in, he had a bottle on the counter waiting for me.

I didn't think I was an alcoholic. I thought I drank every day because I wanted to and it relaxed me. I thought I could stop anytime I wanted. It was like the drugs that I was using. I thought I could quit any time I wanted. I had always thought I could quit doing anything any time I wanted. That is, except cocaine. The queen had my number the first time I shot it, and I knew it.

That is how many alcoholics are. They don't think they have a problem. That is why they don't attend Alcoholics Anonymous meetings. They don't think they need it. They don't think they are alcoholics. Even if they do attend a meeting, they can't bring themselves to say what people in the meetings normally say. "Hello. My name is -----. I'm an alcoholic."

Chemical dependency runs in families. Studies have shown that more than half of all alcoholics have, or had, at least one alcoholic parent. Current research confirms that both genetics and environment play important roles in determining how substances becomes dependent.

I believe alcoholism and other addictions do run, for the most part, in families. Mine was no different. As I stated earlier, I came from a long line of alcoholics. I don't think my grandfather knew the affect that he was having on me when I was sitting on the bar stool next to him in Jack's Foxhole.

Early use is linked with chemical dependency. According to a recent study by the National Institute on Alcohol Abuse and Alcoholism, people who begin drinking before the age of 15 are four times more likely to have problems than people who begin at 21.

I left the ministry and the church when I was 20 years old. I was a dope fiend for most of twenty-two years, from 1969 to 1991, and an alcoholic until 1993. In 1994, I went back to church and back to preaching the Gospel and I was doing quite well, for a while.

I moved to Greensboro, North Carolina to go into business with a friend of mine. One day, I attended a birthday party in his backyard and drank a glass of after-dinner wine along with the other guests. There is nothing wrong with having a little glass of wine, is there? Maybe not for most people, but I had been an alcoholic for almost 25 years. That innocent little glass of wine woke something inside me. Before I knew it, I was in the kitchen with a wine bottle turned upside down. After that, it was like I had never quit drinking.

Needless to say, the business failed and I returned to St. Louis. When I got back, I became a "closet drinker." I was too ashamed to let anybody know that I had a problem and needed help. I had too much pride. After all, I was Rev. Barr. I was in charge of the substance abuse ministry. I couldn't let people know that I was drinking again. So, after church was over and I wanted to go to a liquor store, I would change my clothes so I didn't look like a preacher.

I stopped going to liquor stores because I didn't want anyone to see me going in or coming out. I went to gas stations that sold liquor. One night, I went to the gas station that was down the street from my apartment in Ferguson, Missouri.

I stood in line, waiting my turn so I could buy my booze, but at the last minute, I changed my mind and decided not to buy it. I was tired of living a double life and decided try to quit again. I bought something from behind the counter and turned to leave the store. Just then, the young lady who was standing in line behind me said hello. Then she said, "You don't remember me do you?" I looked at her for a few seconds, trying to recognize her. She smiled and said, "You baptized me yesterday."

That really messed me up. When I got to my car, I just sat there crying. Supposed I hadn't changed my mind and ordered that half pint. What would that have done to her? What would that have done to her faith in God and her respect for preachers? I wish I could say I quit drinking after my encounter with the young lady. I can't.

Because of my reputation and my pride, I didn't seek the help that I needed. I didn't want anyone to know that I wasn't perfect and I had a weakness, so instead of talking to someone, I preached sermons like: "The Closet", "Super Saints" and "I've Fallen, and I Can't Get Up." No one knew that when I was preaching those sermons, I was talking about myself.

I don't know why God allowed me to struggle with alcohol for so long. Maybe He wanted me to know that I hadn't "arrived" and I wasn't the "great" Rev. Burton Barr Jr. that people were telling me that I was. Or maybe it was because I didn't have true compassion for alcoholics.

To be honest, I had more respect for thieves, murderers and drug addicts than I did for alcoholics. There were times that I didn't even want to be around my own brother because of his drinking. So I couldn't let anyone know that I was drinking too. I was too ashamed.

My drinking had gotten to the point that I started making bad choices and doing stupid things. Things that could have cost me my reputation, my ministry and even my life, but I thank God for His grace and mercy. I thank Him for friends who noticed that I was doing some things that were uncharacteristic of me. They wouldn't leave me alone until they got to the bottom of it. Then they loved me with the love of Jesus Christ.

I often wondered how I was able to overcome heroin and cocaine but alcohol was kicking my behind. I finally took the advice of some of my friends and went to treatment. Don't get me wrong, I am not downplaying the controlling power of heroin and cocaine. I anticipated that. The problem was, I underestimated the treacherous and cunning power of alcohol. It caught me completely off guard. I didn't expect that tough of a fight.

When I was in the Marines, I did a little boxing for a brief time. During one of my fights, my opponent gave me all that I could handle and then some. Since he was smaller than me, I thought I was going to have an easy victory. Nothing was further from the truth.

We went toe to toe during the entire fight. When the final round was about to begin, my corner man said I was ahead on points. To win the fight, all I had to do was keep fighting until the bell rings.

That was the longest round that I had ever fought. I think my opponent turned into Popeye and his corner man gave him some spinach before the last round started. I was hitting him with everything I had but my punches didn't faze him.

His punches felt like giant boulders, coming from every direction. I was ready to quit but I kept hearing my corner man yelling, "Keep fighting until the bell rings." I was thinking to myself, "When is the bell going to ring?" When the fight was over, I found out that I had barely won. That was my third and final fight.

Some of our battles that we thought were going to be easy, turns out to be the toughest battles we've ever had. You go in thinking, "I can handle it. I got this. I can quit any time I want." That was the attitude I had about alcohol.

I never went to treatment for heroin or cocaine, not for real. When I went, it was just to fool some people or to get myself out of trouble. I attended the mandatory classes and sessions, but my heart and mind wasn't in it. Remind me to come back to that.

When I was in treatment for alcohol, I was talking with another one of the patients, in between sessions. He told me what his drug of choice was, then asked me about mine. When I told him it was alcohol, he turned to me with a puzzled look on his face and said, "Is that all?"

When we were in group sessions, I saw that same expression on people's faces when I talked about my battle with alcohol. They looked at me as if they were saying, "You are here for that?"

They looked at alcoholism the same way that I had. It is not that big of a problem. It was like the guy that I fought in the ring during my last fight; a lightweight. They were fighting the big fights. Heroin. Crack. Meth. Fentanyl.

I had fought heroin and won. I had fought cocaine and won. I had fought crack and won. Now I was going toe to toe with an opponent that I had underestimated. I was ahead on points, because I realized I needed help. Now, all I had to do was keep fighting until the bell rang.

That is something that everyone in recovery has to do. Fight. It does not matter what your drug of choice is. Fight. It does not matter how many times you have been knocked down. Fight. It does not matter who has given up on you. Fight. Keep fighting until the bell rings.

I have said many times that I never went to treatment or rehab for my drug addiction. That is true, but I got some of the knowledge and benefits of rehab when I was there as a sham.

Let me try to explain this. I have been doing prison ministry for more than 25 years. During some of the church services where I was preaching or teaching, there were inmates that sat in the back of the room, not paying attention. They didn't want to be there, instead, they just wanted to get out of their cells for a while. After being there, week after week or month after month, they started taking in some of the things that were being said. I didn't know that was what happened to me. Although I was deep in my addiction, there were times when I remembered something that was said while sitting in the back of the room in treatment.

So don't give up on your child. Don't give up on your spouse. Don't give up on your niece or nephew, or cousin. Don't preach at them or talk down to them. Talk to them. Let them know you love them and you are there for them, but don't enable them because they will try you.

In the Big Book of Alcoholics Anonymous, one of the first things that people learn in the meetings, are the twelve steps. There are different versions of the steps. But all of them have the same basic meaning and they all have the same key word. Powerless. That is what all alcoholics must realize before they can start to recover. They are powerless when it comes to alcohol.

Everyone is powerless to something. It could be men, women, food, cigarettes, money or sex. I don't care how smart or how strong you are. Something has your number.

Brian Cavanaugh told the story about an important football game. One team was much larger than the other.

The coach for the smaller team realized his team was not able to contain or block the larger team, so he decided to call plays that went to Calhoun, the fastest back in the area.

The coach told his quarterback to give the ball to Calhoun and let him run with it. The team ran the first play, but Calhoun did not get the ball. The second play was again signaled for Calhoun, but again, Calhoun did not get the ball. Now the game was in the final seconds. The smaller team's only hope was for Calhoun to break free and score the winning touchdown.

The team ran the third play, but again Calhoun did not get the ball. The coach was very upset. They were facing the fourth and final play of the game. Again, the coach sent in the play that was designed for Calhoun to run the ball. The ball was snapped, but the quarterback was sacked. The game ended without Calhoun ever touching the ball.

The coach was furious with the quarterback. He said, "I told you four times to give the ball to Calhoun. Now we have lost the game. Why didn't you give the ball to Calhoun?" The quarterback said, "I tried to give the ball to Calhoun four times. The problem was, Calhoun didn't want the ball."

There are a lot of opportunities and programs available for people who are dealing with addictions. Some of the addicts have loving families. There are support systems in place. All they have to do is accept the help what is being offered to them.

In the above story, everything had been laid out for Calhoun. The coach called the play for him to get the ball. The quarterback tried to hand him the ball. The front line was in place to block for him. All Calhoun had to do was take the ball and run with it. The problem was, Calhoun didn't want the ball.

There are so many people who have everything that they need to be successful in overcoming their addictions. A bed is being held for them at the rehab center. There is someone who will take them to the center. The ball is there for them to take it and run. The problem is, they don't want the ball. They are not really ready.

In his book, Alcohol and the Christian Influence, C. Aubrey Hearn told a true story about an advertising man in New York City who thought of an idea that would make him a large commission. He called on his prospect and told him the plans. The prospect warmed up to the proposal. A luncheon date was set to clinch the deal.

The advertising man, who liked to drink, decided to celebrate. So he took a drink before the conference. One drink led to another. When he arrived for the luncheon, he was smashed. His behavior was unruly, ill-tempered and insulting. The deal was quickly called off. An important business contract was lost because the salesman could not stay away from the bottle.

Some people, when they are talking about substances, they say drugs and alcohol. When telling their story, someone might say, "I was on drugs and alcohol for years." If you haven't noticed, I say the same thing sometimes.

The truth is, alcohol is a drug. According to drugfreeworld.org, it is classed as a depressant. That means it slows down the vital functions. Some of the results are slurred speech, unsteady movement, disturbed perception and an inability to react quickly. It affects the mind by reducing a person's ability to think rationally and distorts his or her judgment.

Alcohol dependence consists of four symptoms:

1) **Craving**: A strong need or compulsion to drink.
2) **Loss of control**: The inability to limit one's drinking on any given occasion.
3) **Physical dependence**: Withdrawal symptoms such as nausea, sweating, shakiness and anxiety occur when alcohol use is stopped after a period of heavy drinking.
4) **Tolerance**: The need to drink greater amounts of alcohol in order to get high.

An increasingly heavy drinker often says he can stop whenever he chooses. He just never chooses to do so. Drugfreeworld.org goes on to say, alcoholism is not a destination. It is a progression. It is a long road of deterioration in which life continuously worsens.

It is not always easy to understand why people drink. C. Aubrey Hearn suggested that some of the reasons might be psychological while others were practical. In his book, "Alcohol and Christian Influence", he mentions seven examples that stood out to him. However, based on my own personal experience, these examples take on a slightly different meaning:

1) **To heighten self-esteem**: Some people are naturally shy, timid or self-conscious. Alcohol releases inhibitions that allow a shy person to open up.

2) **To remove tension and anxiety**: Many people are overwhelmed by the storms that come about in their lives. Drinking helps them relax, forget their problems and not be bothered by the storm.

3) **Pleasure**: To some people, pleasure is everything. They crave physical satisfaction and gratification and alcohol serves to enhance this desire.

4) **To remove guilt**: Alcohol can provide a temporary bandage to cover the guilt that people hold onto. Alcohol can also numb the pain that the bandage can't cover.

5) **Courage**: We used to call alcohol, "Liquid Courage." Sometimes people drink to summon courage to commit sin or do something they would not ordinarily do.

6) **Curiosity**: For a lot of people, especially young people, trying alcohol satisfies a curiosity. The need to satisfy every curiosity is a slippery slope that I do not recommend.

7) **Social pressure**: Some people drink because others do it, while others drink because others expect them too. The need to "fit in" will be the demise of many of my brothers and sisters.

When I was a child, we had a family dog named Rex. Although Rex was kind of temperamental, I loved playing with him. There were two things that Rex did not allow anyone to do, no matter who they were. First of all, he didn't let anyone stick his or her hand in his doghouse while he was in there. I guess he figured, since we wouldn't let him in our house, we couldn't go in his.

The other thing was, he didn't want anyone to touch his food while he was eating. Everyone in our family knew this and our parents constantly warned Ralph and me.

One day, Ralph and I were playing with a stick on our back porch and we accidentally dropped it. It fell off of the porch and landed in the middle of some food that Rex was eating. Ralph thought he could grab the stick before Rex could grab his hand. Rex growled but Ralph tried it anyway. Bad move. Rex had Ralph's hand before he even got close to the stick!

Ralph ran away crying, so I tried to comfort him by telling him that he went at it the wrong way. I told him to stand back and watch me get the stick. I knew better than to put my hand near Rex's food, so I decided to kick the stick away and then pick it up. Rex growled at me and like Ralph, I decided to try it anyway. Bad move. Rex had my foot before it got close to the stick. Both of us went in the house, crying!

That is how alcohol is to alcoholics. We know we shouldn't mess with it. We tried it before and we got bitten. Instead of learning our lesson, we tried to be slick about that thing.

Ralph and I knew what Rex's rule was, "Don't mess with his food." That is the rule that alcohol has for alcoholics. Don't mess with it. Problem is, we alcoholics do things we know we shouldn't. Maybe we think we can get away with it or it might just be to impress someone. If we simply did what God told us and stayed away from things we know we should avoid, it would spare us a lot of pain in the end.

One of the reasons I wanted to quit drinking was I didn't want to look how some of the people that I saw in the liquor stores looked. I know that might be a vain reason, but it is true. However, that didn't stop me from drinking; it just reminded me of how I was going to look one day if I didn't quit.

I began to ask myself the question quite frequently, "What is so happy about happy hour?" We avoid the rush-hour traffic by sitting in bars for a couple of hours, drinking with coworkers and then getting in our cars and driving home.

Drinking and driving wasn't that big of a deal in the 70's and 80's. People did it all the time. We rode around with can holders in the side windows for our cars for our beer. Like the coke spoons had been acceptable in the 70s, driving around with open cans of beer was acceptable.

I was driving home from work one night when I ran into Coleman. He was one to the older boys from my neighborhood when I was growing up. As children and teenagers, they were the ones that we always wanted to impress.

He had just bought a sandwich and we stopped at a liquor store and bought a fifth of Johnny Walker Red.

While I was driving, Coleman opened the bottle and threw the top out the window. That was a whole fifth of scotch. If the police pulled us over, there was nothing that I could do with the bottle. I couldn't even put it under the seat.

I was trying to be cool and act like that didn't bother me. Obviously it didn't bother Coleman. He took a bite of his sandwich and washed it down with a few swallows of scotch like the cowboys do in the movies.

While we were riding, we drank the entire bottle and talked about old times. I dropped Coleman off at his house and drove home. I have no idea how I got there. I just remember waking up the next morning with a terrible hangover.

When I was a teenager, most of my friends were a year or so older than me. I looked up to them the way we all looked up to Coleman and the boys that were his age.

After school one day, my friend, Joe and I were riding home on the bus. I was a freshman, Joe was a sophomore. There were no school buses back then. Students rode public transportation. My friends and I always sat in the back of the buses so we could smoke.

Since Joe was older than me and I was new to the high school thing, I took my cue from him. We were sitting near the back with the window open while we were smoking. Joe was next to the window. I sat next to the aisle. I felt someone nudge my foot. When I looked around, I saw a very big white gentleman standing next to me. He said, "Put it out."

Joe was looking out of the window, so he didn't see the man. So I nudged Joe and said, "He said, 'Put it out.'" Joe just said, "Screw him" and kept looking out the window. I felt another nudge on my foot. When I looked around again I saw the same man. This time he was holding a badge. I nudged Joe again. I said, "He got a badge, Joe." We both threw our cigarettes out the window.

Teenagers oftentimes take their cues from their peers. The pressure of their peers makes them want to be accepted. They want to be liked. They want to fit in and be one of the crowd. They want to be cool so they start smoking because everyone else is doing it. They start drinking because everyone else is doing it. Everything they do starts to be because everyone else is doing it.

Unfortunately, it is not just teenagers that get caught up in peer pressure. I've seen a lot of adults fall into that trap as well. They start doing things or trying things because they want to impress someone. Usually it is a woman or man that they are attracted to, or new friends that they are hanging with. Sometimes they're curious and they want to try something, but they end up liking it a little too much.

My mother, father, Ralph and I were sitting at the

kitchen table one evening, eating dinner. Mother and Ralph were eating chitterlings (chitlins). Dad and I were eating chicken because neither one of us liked chitterlings. While we were eating, Ralph was crying. He was just eating and crying. That went on for quite a while.

Finally, my mother asked Ralph what was wrong with him. He said, "I don't want to eat these." Mother said, "Then get some chicken. You don't have to eat that." Ralph looked at her, still crying and said, "But they taste good."

That is the problem that many of us have with our drug of choice. We don't want to drink anymore, but it tastes good. We don't want to smoke crack anymore, but it feels good. We don't want to shoot heroin anymore, but it makes us feel good.

I've heard people say, "Everything that's good to you, is not good for you." Nevertheless, we go after it. That's been the root of many of life's problems. It tastes good. It feels good. She looks good. He makes me feel good.

Like many others, I made some really bad choices when I was drinking. Some of them were outright dumb. Like the time I was so drunk, I bumped into several tables when I was leaving a club. I got in my car and drove home. The next day, someone asked me why I drove in that condition. I replied, "I was too drunk to walk!"

I always stopped and got a half pint when I got off from work. I would sit in the parking lot, gulp it down, and drive off. One night I was having trouble with my car. My head lights kept flickering. I stopped at Walgreens and got my usual bottle. I sat in the parking lot, contemplating whether if I should drink it at the moment, or wait until I got home.

With my head lights flickering, I knew there was a greater chance of me getting pulled over. What made it worst was, I lived down the street from the Ferguson police station. I had to drive past there to get home. After giving it careful thought for a minute, I turned the bottle up and drank it. Then I drove off.

I pull into the parking lot of my apartment building and got out of the car. Just then, a Ferguson police officer pulled up. He didn't get out of his car. He said he noticed my lights flashing and ask if I was okay. I said I was and went inside. He probably thought I was signaling him because I was in trouble or needed help. I needed help alright. Big time.

Some years ago I broke my foot while loading a truck with some donations for one of the ministries of the church. I was off work for some time. After several weeks, I was finally able to return to church, but I was on crutches. So, I sat on the first bench that I could get to. It was the bench that was closest to the door.

After a few weeks, I realized that everyone that sat on that particular bench was crippled in one way or another. I came in on crutches, someone else came in sitting in a wheelchair, another used a walker and someone else rode in on a scooter.

One Sunday, a new lady came in on a walker. She looked around, in search of a seat but the bench was full. Just then, the brother that was sitting next to me got up, escorted the lady to his seat and he moved to another bench. When I looked around the church, I realized that there were people all over the sanctuary that had sat on that bench at one time or another, but now, they are sitting on other benches. Some of them were sitting in the pulpit. Some of them were sitting in the choir stand. Some of them were sitting on the usher's bench. And some of them were sitting on the bench with the deacons.

The world is full of people who are crippled. Some of them are crippled by alcohol. Some of them are crippled by drugs. Some of them are crippled by depression. Some of them are crippled by hopelessness.

All of us have been crippled and broken at some point in our lives. Then one day some of us finally realized that we needed help, so we took a seat on the cripple's bench. We stayed there on that bench until we were ready to move on and take our place in society. Too many people are still sitting there. Instead of reaching out and trying to help someone else, they have become comfortable, just sitting on the bench with the crippled folks.

It might look like I am spending more time on the subject of alcoholism than on any other subject. I am. Alcohol has ruined more families, destroyed more careers and damaged more lives than any other drug. It is cunning and deceitful. Some people don't realize how harmful it is because it is legal. Don't get me wrong. I am not saying alcohol should be banned. A lot of people enjoy it and they drink responsibly, however, our young people should be educated about the potential risks that come along with it.

I've made a lot of bad choices while under the influence of alcohol and I thank God the outcomes didn't turn out as badly as they could have. By the grace of God, I've never received a DUI or DWI and I've never caused an accident.

If there were statistics about how many people were in accidents while driving after leaving happy hour, what would they look like? Also, look at the bars and clubs at closing time. The DJ says, "You don't have to go home, but you have to leave here." Where do they go? To their cars. More than 10,000 people are killed each year by drunk drivers. Organizations like "Mothers Against Drunk Driving" are doing fantastic work, combating this problem.

During this writing, the world is in the middle of the COVID-19 pandemic. People are dying because many of us are not taking it seriously. Drug addiction is a pandemic in this country and people are dying because we are not taking it seriously. Alcoholism is a pandemic in this country as well and people are also dying because we are not taking it seriously.

There are, however, some people who are taking it very seriously, trying their best and doing all they can to break free from the bondage of addiction. They are crying out for help. They have called the rehab centers, but there are no beds available. They tried other places, but they don't have insurance. Their family and friends have given up on them. I want to encourage you to just do your best, then trust in the Lord to do the rest. Don't give up. Don't give in. Keep fighting until the bell rings.

Smoke Gets In Your Eyes

The way society views marijuana has drastically changed in recent years. Not only is it no longer illegal in some states, but some jurisdictions have stores or shops where it can be sold. It has become a big business.

For years, selling and possessing marijuana were criminal offences, resulting in countless men and women being arrested and jailed all across the country. Marijuana is not the innocent drug that some of us think it is. For years it has been described as the gateway drug. Now, I'm not suggesting that everyone who smokes weed will end up shooting heroin or smoking crack or meth, but the fact is, most of the people who are using hard drugs started by smoking weed.

Most of the people who smoke or have smoked marijuana started when they were teenagers, some were even younger. Peer pressure and curiosity may have played a major role. For years, marijuana was a very popular drug.

That popularity may have increased in the70s. Those were the wild child years in America. The country was changing. People were protesting various issues.

Young people rebelled against many of the ideas and philosophies of their parents. They grew their hair longer and traded in their buttoned down suits and Ivy League clothes for bell bottoms, t-shirts, dashikis and flip flops.

People opposed the Vietnam war. They turned to disco, peace signs and free love. African Americans were becoming more interested in their heritage. Women were burning their bras and demanding equal rights and young America chose marijuana instead of cocktails.

I stopped hanging out with my friends and got involved in the church when I was 16 years old. Before I left, our idea of fun was house parties, playing basketball in the alley, spending time with our girlfriends and drinking beer on the weekends.

I was licensed and ordained to preach when I was seventeen, but I left the church and returned to the streets when I was 20 years old. A lot of things had changed. My friends were no longer teenagers. Another thing that had changed was everyone was smoking marijuana.

I had never smoked weed before. I had never even seen a joint but eventually, I started smoking it too. Like so many others, I tried it because of peer pressure. Everyone that I was with was smoking it. I didn't want them to think I wasn't cool, so when they passed me the joint, I took it. They probably knew that was my first time smoking anyway because when I took a hit I started coughing like crazy. I tried to play it off but I think they knew.

Everyone that I knew smoked weed. It was the thing to do. It was not like the hard drugs. No one was getting hooked on it. At lease, I didn't think so.

I was in the Marines for almost five years. Well, some of that time didn't really count. I had been kicked out with a bad conduct discharge. So, although I was no longer in the Marines, my discharge wasn't official for several months.

We smoked a lot of weed when I was in the Marines. They didn't test people like they do now. One night, while I was walking guard duty, I decided to take a break and get high. I saw, what looked like, a large metal crate. I sat on it and lit a joint and a cigarette.

When I finished smoking the joint, I stood up and reached for my rifle. When I bent down, I noticed a sign that was on the side of the crate. It was too dark out there for me to see what it said, so I lit the cigarette lighter so I could see it better. It said, "DANGER. NO SMOKING WITHIN 500 FEET."

I closed the cigarette lighter and started moving away from the crate but I was so high, all I could do was laugh. That's an example of some of the bad choices we make when we are stoned. I had always heard that God watches over fools and babies. I wasn't a baby, but He was surely watching over me!

I had always thought I would never quit smoking marijuana. I envisioned myself heading to the local dealer on my walker when I was 90 years old. I had always smoked weed. As far as I was concerned, that was just a part of life. I remember when I wouldn't let people smoke cigarettes in my car. They could only smoke weed.

According to the American Addiction Center, marijuana is one of the most popular drugs on the market today. While it may have the impression of being a harmless, fun substance, it is still a drug that changes what goes on in the mind, sometimes with significant consequences. The long-term effects on the brain and body make marijuana a dangerous drug to a lot of people, leading to negative outcomes that don't show until years later.

The National Institute of Drug Abuse says marijuana is the most commonly used psychotropic drug in the United States, after alcohol. Its use is widespread among young people. In 2018, more than 11.8 million young adults used marijuana in the past year. According to the Monitoring the Future Survey, rates of past year marijuana use among middle and high school students have remained steady, but the number of teens in 8th and 10th grades who say they use it daily have increased.

With the growing popularity of vaping devices,

teens have started vaping Tetrahydrocannabinol (Don't ask me how to pronounce it). Tetrahydrocannabinol is known as THC, the ingredient in marijuana that produces the high. Nearly 4% of 12th graders saying they vape THC daily. In addition, the number of young people who believe regular marijuana use is risky is decreasing.

When I was a teenager, I ran with a Chicago street gang named, "The Roman Saints." I wasn't really a member. Dad didn't play that. I just hung with them sometimes. Maybe I was a "wanna be".

One day, some of us were hanging out on the corner when we spotted several members of the Vice Lords. We started chasing them down Roosevelt Road. I had always been a fast runner. As a matter of fact, I prided myself in being able to outrun most people.

I was new to this gang thing and I wanted to impress the guys that I was with. So, while we were chasing the Vice Lords, I decided to show them my speed and ability. Naturally, I was ahead of everyone else. After several blocks, the Vice Lords stopped running. I said to myself, "We got them now." Then I noticed that they had not only stopped running. They were just standing there, looking at me as if they were waiting for me.

When I turned to see where the rest of the gang members were, I got the shock of my life. They were standing on one of the corners, about a block and a half behind me, yelling for me to come back. All of a sudden, the Vice Lords that I had been chasing were chasing me.

More of them joined in the chase, cutting off my escape route. I ended up getting one of the worst beat-downs in my life. I found out that there was a street that we did not cross. That street was the dividing line that entered into their territory.

There is a line that divides casual use from addiction. It is not clear where that line is, but far too many people have crossed it. Most of them didn't even know that there is a line. They were just chasing their drug of choice.

They were feeling good and enjoying themselves like they always had. Suddenly, they were in unfamiliar territory. They have crossed the line. Now they are facing one of the worst beat-downs of their lives.

Marijuana is smoked in various ways. Besides the traditional method of rolling it in tobacco paper, some people smoke blunts. That is when you take some or all of the tobacco out of a cigar and replace it with marijuana. Sometimes it is mixed with cocaine. That may have changed in some variation over the years. I have been out of the game for a while.

There were no blunts when I was getting high. Sometimes we used pipes, bongs (water pipes), holders and rolling paper. When the joint got short, we used roach clips, but that's ancient history.

Some addicts smoke PCP, also known as angel dust among other names. PCP is a drug used for its mind-altering effects. It may cause hallucinations, distorted perceptions of sounds and violent behavior. As a recreational drug, it is typically smoked, but may be taken by mouth, snorted, or injected. It may also be mixed with marijuana or tobacco.

While usage peaked in the 1970s, between 2005 and 2011 an increase in visits to emergency rooms as a result of the drug occurred. As of 2017 about 1% of people in grade twelve reported using PCP in the prior year while 2.9% of those over the age of 25 reported using it at some point in their life.

Other names for PCP use are Sherman sticks, happy sticks, dippers and water. Sherman sticks is a Sherman cigarette that is dipped in PCP or "water." Happy sticks are marijuana cigarettes that are dipped. I have heard and read that the water the cigarettes are dipped in is formaldehyde (embalming fluid).

Smoking water made people do some strange things. The first time that I heard of it was when Ralph called me at work one evening and was told my cousins were tearing up their mother's house. When I got there, I found out they had smoked a Sherman stick.

Having the drug using nature that I have, I had to

try it. What I didn't realize was my addiction had progressed to the point where my perception of reality was distorted and my judgment was so impaired, it seemed reasonable to go on and do that.

After all, I had tried almost every drug that I had heard of or encountered at the time. Why should Sherman sticks be any different? When a heroin addict overdoses, other addicts want to know where they copped the drugs from. They don't believe it will happen to them. Well, I didn't tear up my house, but I did scare my mother to death. She was living with me at the time.

Ralph and I started smoking Sherman sticks quite often. Most of the time, it was uneventful; just an intense high. One time we were at his lady friend's house. She didn't like us smoking there, so we walked around the corner and sat on a bench at the bus stop. After we smoked the dipper, we couldn't find our way back to her house. You'd think that would've been our wakeup call but after that happened a couple of times, instead of quitting, we made a game out of it.

Some of the experiences were not so funny. Like the time we bought a dipper and smoked it in the car. I had backed into a parking space on a hill so no one could sneak up behind us.

After we finished smoking, I put the car in reverse and stepped on the gas. We started going backwards. I hit the brakes, checked the gear shift to make sure it was in reverse and stepped on the gas again. We started going backwards again. I hit the brakes again. Ralph asked what was wrong. I said, "The car keeps going backwards." I checked the gear shift again. I made sure it was in reverse. I stepped on the gas again. You guessed it. The car went backwards again. Ralph hollered, "Hey man. Don't do that no more. We're gonna go over that hill." I said, "I don't know what's wrong with this car. I keep putting it in reverse, but it keeps going backwards!"

Sometime later, I moved back to Chicago. Ralph eventually moved back too. Dippers were not called Sherman sticks there. They were called happy sticks. We continued occasionally smoking sticks. One night, Ralph must have smoked too much.

I was standing in the living room at the kitchen table, reading a newspaper when I heard a weird noise in the living room. Ralph walked into the kitchen and had a strange look on his face. He said he was going to kill me. I said, "What's wrong with you? I'm your brother!" He replied, "You ain't my brother, you're the devil MF'er and I'm going to kill you!" He started walking towards me as I moved around the kitchen table, calling his name. After a few seconds, he snapped out of it and didn't remember any of it.

The straw that broke the camel's back for me was

the night that I finally was able to get some alone time with a beautiful woman named Lisa. I had been trying to get with her for weeks and she was finally in my room with me, smoking crack and happy sticks.

We were getting ready to go to bed when I decided to get some beers for us from the refrigerator. I went in the kitchen and opened the refrigerator door. The next thing I knew, I was on top of the refrigerator and Lisa was walking out the door. I never smoked water again.

I have never smoked crystal meth and don't know anyone who has, but according to Medical News Today, crystal meth is a highly addictive, illegal stimulant drug that has a long-lasting euphoric effect. Known informally as meth, ice, or glass, it resembles shiny "rocks" or fragments of glass of varying sizes. It is known more formally as crystal methamphetamine.

The drug is odorless and colorless. It is made in illegal labs, often by combining ingredients derived from over-the-counter drugs with toxic substances. The Drug Policy Alliance maintains that 11 million Americans, on at least one occasion, have tried methamphetamine.

Crystal meth is popular among young adults at dance clubs and parties. It is taken for its euphoric effects. Some people take it because it can lead to rapid weight loss, although most of the lost weight tends to return when a person stops using the drug.

The body also gradually becomes tolerant to crystal meth, reducing the weight-loss effect over time. Some people prefer crystal meth to other illicit drugs because the sense of euphoria it gives can last for up to 12 hours. This is a much longer duration than cocaine, a drug with similar effects.

People with depression may choose to take crystal meth for its mood-enhancing properties. Others may be attracted by the increased libido and sexual pleasure often associated with this drug.

I smoked a lot of weed back in the day. One of the bad things about smoking so much weed is, it affects your memory. I was going to say something else, but I forgot what it was. So I'm going to stop here.

Burton Barr Jr.

The Man on the Side of the Road

--- † ---

In the 10th chapter of the book of Luke, Jesus told a story that is known as, "The Good Samaritan."

²⁵ And behold, a certain lawyer stood up and tested Him, saying, *"Teacher, what shall I do to inherit eternal life?"*

²⁶ He said to him, *"What is written in the law? What is your reading of it?"*

²⁷ So he answered and said, *"You shall love the Lord your God with all your heart, with all your soul, with all your strength, and with all your mind,* and *your neighbor as yourself."*

²⁸ And He said to him, *"You have answered rightly; do this and you will live."*

²⁹ But he, wanting to justify himself, said to Jesus, *"And who is my neighbor?"*

³⁰ Then Jesus answered and said: *"A certain man went*

down from Jerusalem to Jericho, and fell among thieves, who stripped him of his clothing, wounded him, and departed, leaving him half dead.

[31] Now by chance a certain priest came down that road. And when he saw him, he passed by on the other side.

[32] Likewise a Levite, when he arrived at the place, came and looked, and passed by on the other side.

[33] But a certain Samaritan, as he journeyed, came where he was. And when he saw him, he had compassion.

[34] So he went to him and bandaged his wounds, pouring on oil and wine; and he set him on his own animal, brought him to an inn, and took care of him.

[35] On the next day, when he departed, he took out two denarii, gave them to the innkeeper, and said to him, 'Take care of him; and whatever more you spend, when I come again, I will repay you.'

[36] So which of these three do you think was neighbor to him who fell among the thieves?"

[37] And he said, "He who showed mercy on him." Then Jesus

said to him, "Go and do likewise." (NKJV)

In the story, Jesus talked about the misfortune of a young man who chose a dangerous road to travel on. The road from Jerusalem to Jericho was notorious for its danger and difficulty. There are some who might fault the young man for his predicament. If he hadn't been on that road, he wouldn't have been beaten and left lying there.

That is how some people feel about the men and women who are addicted. Even the ones who are trying their best to overcome their addictions and are looking for help. Some of our respectable citizens, including some of our church members, look down on them and turn their heads like the priest and the Levite. They just shake their heads and leave them lying on the side of the road.

They say it's the addict's fault. They shouldn't have started messing with that stuff in the first place. There are some who overcame their addictions. Now, instead of reaching out and offering words of encouragement, they look down their noses at the ones who are still struggling. They forgot that at one time, they too were lying on the side of the road.

When I was in prison, I read a book about a famous gangster named, Lucky Luciano. He was a crime boss in New York in the 1920s and 30s. He was like the godfather in the movie. His organization controlled the gambling, bootlegging, prostitution and many other illegal activities.

According to the book, one of his lieutenants, Meyer Lansky, came to him with the idea of trafficking heroin. He talked about how much money that would bring in.

Luciano thought dealing in something as detestable as heroin would bring major repercussion from government officials and turn the public against them. He said the money that they would make was not worth it, but Lansky was persistent. He said, "All we have to do is put it in the (N-word) neighborhoods and let them sell it to each other." The inner cities are inundated with drug houses and liquor stores, but addictions know no boundaries. It will conquer people of any race, age, gender or nationality.

When I was a child, people would ask me what I wanted to be when I grew up. Not once did I say I wanted to be a junkie. I never said I wanted be a slave to a needle or a pipe. I never said I want to be one of the children of the night.

No child dreamed of being a thief, a robber or a prostitute so they can support their habit. No one knew what they were signing up for when they took their first hit, their first snort or their first shot.

I was told that one of the prisons in Missouri had a sign at the end of a hall where all of the new prisoners had to pass through. It said, "**Leave all of your hopes and dreams behind.**"

That sign should be posted at the entrance of every dope house, every crack house, every shooting gallery and on every corner where drugs are sold.

People start using drugs for different reasons. I listed some of them earlier but one of the main reasons that some people start using has been the down fall of many. It is the people that they choose to associate with. It is the people that they call their friends.

My father tried to tell me that. He said, "Son. That crowd you're running with don't mean you no good." But I wouldn't listen to him. I said, "Dad. You don't know what you're talking about. These are my friends!"

I found out that he was right, because it wasn't long before I ended up in the Cook County Jail in Chicago. I sat there wondering, "Where are my friends now?"

When the guards were passing out the mail, they just walked past my cell because I didn't even have a letter. I sat there wondering, "Where are my friends now?"

On visiting days, I wanted somebody to come and see me. I just sat there, trying to pretend I wasn't hurting when my number wasn't called because no one cared enough to visit me. I just sat there in my cell, fighting back the tears and wondering, "Where are my friends now?"

Sometimes I would think about all of the money that I had thrown away on drugs, alcohol and wild parties, trying to buy somebody's friendship. Now, no one would even send me a dime so I could buy a bar of soap to wash my face. All I could do was sit there wondering, "Where are my friends now?"

People are hurting. One day, they walked down Drug Road. They had no idea just how dangerous it was. Along the way, they were attacked and beaten. They were beaten by heroin. They were beaten by cocaine. Beaten by crack. Beaten by meth. Beaten by alcohol. Beaten by pills. They are lying on the side of the road, beaten and bruised.

There's a man on the side of the road that needs you. Tear yourself away from the television or the computer or the golf course long enough to do something to bless him. He's homeless and hopeless because of his addiction. He needs somebody to help him. Pour some oil and wine in his wounds and bandage up his brokenness.

There's a woman on the side of the road that needs you. She's selling her body because her habit has her bound. Or maybe some pimp has her in his clutches and won't let her go free. Go see about her. Pour some oil and wine in her wounds and bandage up her brokenness.

There's a man on the side of the road that needs you. He was strong, athletic and played sports in school but never learned his lessons in class. In fact, he can barely read his own name, so he can't keep a job or support his family. As a result, he turned to alcohol to ease his pain. He needs somebody to come pour some oil and wine in his wounds and bandage up his brokenness.

There are people on the side of the road that need you. They've been to war and stayed there long enough to come back home unable to function like they used to. Fear and distress are their constant companions. Their minds are blown away and now, drugs are their only comfort. They need someone to come pour oil and wine in their wounds and bandage up their brokenness.

Can you see them? Some of them aren't strangers. They're family and friends and co-workers. Can the Lord count on you to pick them up from the side of road?

Jesus said, "When you have done this to the least of these my brethren you have done it to me."

I was that man on the side of the road. But Jesus sent somebody one day, who poured some oil and wine in my wounds and bandaged up my brokenness. Now I have been redeemed.

Part of this chapter contain excerpts from the sermon, "*Man By The Side Of The Road*", by Dr. Ronald L. Bobo, Sr.

Burton Barr Jr.

121

---------------------- † ----------------------

Psalm 121 has a very special place in my heart; it was one of two Psalms that my father taught me, when I was very young and didn't know anything about the Lord. The first one was the 23rd Psalm. I didn't know God and had no idea how much He loved me. My father wanted me to know just who my shepherd was, so he opened his Bible to the 23rd Psalm and showed me where it says, "The Lord is my Shepherd".

You see, he didn't want me to be confused about this thing. He wanted me to know exactly who my shepherd is. He wanted to make sure that I knew who it is that I was supposed to follow.

He wanted me to know that the neighborhood gang leader was not my shepherd. He wanted me to know that the corner drug dealer was not my shepherd. As much as my father loved me and would do anything for me, he wanted me to know that not even he was my shepherd. So he sat me down one day and said, "Son, the Lord is your shepherd."

When I got older, I backslid. I turned my back on God and walked away from the church. I became an alcoholic with a heroin and cocaine habit that was costing me an average of $200.00 a day. My drug habit led me to a life of crime. I was in and out of trouble and in and out of jails and prisons all across this country. I was living a life that was full of misery and pain. I knew that I was in trouble and I desperately wanted someone to help me, but I didn't know where to go to find the help that I so badly needed.

My father came to me one day. Once again he opened his Bible, but this time it was to Psalm 121. He showed me where it said, "I will lift up my eyes to the hills from whence comes my help. My help comes from the Lord who made heaven and earth."

Then he said, "Son, whenever you need help, just look to the hills and call on the Lord, and if you really mean it, then all you've got to do is just hold on, because help is on the way."

According to the notes in The Life Application Bible, Psalm 121 expresses assurance and hope in God's protection day and night. He not only made hills, but He made heaven and earth as well. We should never trust in a lesser power than God himself. Not only is He all powerful, He also watches over us. Nothing diverts or deters Him. We are safe. We never outgrow our need for God's untiring watch over our lives.

When I was a child, my friends and I couldn't get

away with anything on Christiana because of "The Heads." That was what we called my mother and her friends because their heads were always sticking out of their windows.

All of the houses were either two story flats or three story apartment buildings. So, all up and down the street, there were heads popping in and out of windows all day and late into the night.

We knew they were watching us. Years later, when we matured, we realized they were not just watching us, they were watching over us. That's how God is. He is not just watching us, He is watching over us.

God was watching over me through my years of addiction. When I overdosed and should have died, He was there, watching over me. When I was at the dope houses and the stickup men were holding guns on me, He was watching over me.

When I was in prison, no one messed with me, and it wasn't because I was so "tough". God was watching over me! When I was running the streets, laying, playing and parlaying, any one of those con games could have gotten me killed, but God was there. He was watching over me. When I was walking the streets at night, He was with me.

I will never forget the night that I decided to walk to a drug house late one night. It was well past midnight and the drug house was a little over two miles away. For some reason, I was a little nervous about making the walk that night, but I needed the drugs.

When I started walking, a dog came up from behind me. It startled me at first, but he started walking a few feet from me. Every time that I turned a corner, he turned with me. I didn't know if he would have done anything if someone attacked me, but I felt safe with him there.

When I got to the spot, I said goodbye to the dog, went inside and made my purchase. When I came out, I was surprised to see the dog standing there. He walked with me all the way back home. I was so happy, I decided to get some food for him. I even thought about keeping him, but when I got to my house, he kept walking down the street.

When I got in the house, I started wondering, who was that dog? Why did he walk all that way with me? Could it really have been an angel that God had sent to protect me? Did God instruct him to stay with me until I got home? Was that His way of watching over me that night?

During my years of addiction, there was a period when health and dental care were not high on my list of priorities. Several years after I got clean, one of my teeth was bothering me. The dentist gave me a root canal. Afterwards, she said my teeth needed a deep cleaning.

I was looking forward to it. I thought she was going to polish my teeth with some stuff that tasted like Scope or some other mouth wash. Nothing was further from the truth. I was not prepared for what she did.

It felt like she was digging between my teeth and under my gums with drills, hack saws and screwdrivers. That hurt. It was worse than the root canal. She had the nerve to tell me to come back next week for phase two. I went back, alright. Drunk! I thought the alcohol would dull the pain. It didn't work. It still hurt.

At that time, I was clean from heroin and cocaine but weed and alcohol took a little longer. Some of us come to God so messed up, He has to do a deep cleaning on us from years/decades of addiction, the abuse, hurt and pain that we've endured. We need some deep cleaning. Don't get me wrong, when God saves us, it is instant. However, sometimes in order for us to get to where God wants us to be, He does some deep cleaning and it can be painful.

Some addicts are victims of their environment. On any given day in many of our communities, you will find hundreds of men and women standing idly and aimlessly on city street corners. Such hopelessness will eventually lead to criminal activity, drug use, prison or an early grave.

Our young boys and young girls are witnessing this on a regular basis. They see the hurt. They see the pain. They see the brokenness. They look around and all they see is a world of hopelessness. That is why so many of them have given up before they have even tried.

Not everyone who grew up poor or in the slums or in the projects ended up on drugs or in prison. Many of them overcame their obstacles and did well, but we cannot forget about those who got stuck.

One day, Jesus talked about the end times and who will be with him in paradise.

I was hungry, and you fed me.
I was thirsty, and you gave me a drink.
I was a stranger, and you invited me into your home.
I was naked, and you gave me clothing.
I was sick, and you cared for me.
I was in prison, and you visited me.'

"Then these righteous ones will reply,
'Lord, when did we ever see you hungry and feed you?
Or thirsty and give you something to drink?
Or a stranger and show you hospitality?
Or naked and give you clothing?
When did we ever see you sick or in prison and visit you?'

And the King will say, 'I tell you the truth,
When you did it to one of the least of these
My brothers and sisters,
You were doing it to me!'

Matthew 25:35-40 (NLT)

When I listen to these words of Jesus, this is what I hear:

I was hungry because I lost my job, and you fed me.
I was thirsty because there was no running water in the abandoned building that I lived in, but you gave me a drink.
I was homeless because I got strung out on drugs, but you came to my aid.
I didn't have a coat to wear in this cold weather, but you gave me some clothes.
I was sick and everyone was too busy to see about me, but you cared for me.
I was in prison, but the prison was too far away for my family to visit, but you visited me.
The least of these! The poor - the homeless - the addicts – the alcoholics – the mentally ill – the unemployed – the underemployed – the incarcerated.

A fly was trapped inside of a house. Every day, he looked out of the window and saw all of the other flies just flying around and enjoying themselves in the nice warm sun. He decided that he was going to get out of that house and enjoy the fresh air too.

He flew towards the daylight only to bump his head on the window pane. Again and again he tried to break through, but again and again he bumped his head on the cold, hard glass. He looked in the window seal and saw all of the flies that died trying to escape through the window. He was determined that he was not going to end up like them. He was going to make it to freedom. Unfortunately, after days of trying, he eventually joined all of the other flies that lay dead in the window seal.

The sad thing is, he did not have to die there. Just a few feet from the window was a door that was standing wide open. If he would have chosen the door, he could have flown safely through, but he lay dead in the window seal because he was determined to do it his way.

We are often unsuccessful when we try to break free from situations in our lives because we are determined to do it our way. What we don't realize is there is a door nearby that is standing wide open. Jesus is that door. He is standing there with his arms wide open. He is saying, "I am the way" (John 14:6).

If you are struggling with an addiction, stop trying to kick it your way. Don't end up like the fly. Trust God to work things out His way.

I pray that this book blesses you and that my stories somehow inspire you to get sober. I hope and pray that something that I've said comforts you and brings you peace like Psalm 121 did for me through the years.

Many people believe that scriptures are just words in a book, to be read and memorized. I'm here to tell you that every word of Psalms 121 is real and true. Understanding how to apply these words to my own life was the difference between life and death. Bear with me for a moment as I detail how Psalm 121 is as true and as real as the sky is blue, the grass is green and the water is wet. For updated wording and simplicity, we'll use the New Living Translation:

Psalm 121: 1
I look up to the mountains—
does my help come from there?

During my first month of boot camp, our drill instructors told us about a mountain that we would have to climb. The mountain had a scary name and an even scarier reputation. We were stationed in San Diego, but during our second month we would go to Camp Pendleton for rifle and combat training. That was where the mountain was located.

During the bus ride to Pendleton I convinced myself that the mountain couldn't be that bad. When we got there and I saw it, I found out I was right. It wasn't that bad, it was worse! It looked like the top of it disappeared in the clouds. I was ready to quit and go home.

I looked at that mountain every day for two weeks, terrified. When the day finally came, we got into full combat gear and marched to the trail that was at the foot of the mountain. Then the drill instructor said, "Double time, March!" As we ran further and further up that trail, men started falling out and quitting, but most of us kept going. Then it hit me. I couldn't go any further. I must fall out. I must quit. Just as I was about to stop, I heard the drill instructor say, "Platoon, Halt." I had made it.

When I come up against something that seems impossible to conquer, I think about that mountain. For 22 years of my life, that mountain was my addictions: heroin, cocaine, marijuana, crack, alcohol and sex. By continuing down the trail I was on, I wasn't quitting drugs or any one of my addictions; I was quitting on life. Psalm 121, verse one says, "I look up to the mountains -- does my help come from there?" I compare my "rock bottom" to the valley low of a mountain, but instead of looking up the mountain for help, I found myself on my knees, looking down for my syringe, in an alley. This is why I stayed in my addiction for way longer than I needed to and lost way more than God ever intended for me to lose.

Psalm 121: 2
My help comes from the LORD,
who made heaven and earth!

I had just left a drug house one Sunday morning when I passed a church and heard the sermon about the Prodigal Son. As I sat on the steps, listening to the sermon, I thought about how far I had fallen, how many people I had hurt and how many lives I had destroyed. I started crying and calling out to God, begging Him to forgive me. I felt God telling me to leave Chicago. When I told the other players and hustlers that I was going to leave, they tried to talk me out of it, but my mind was made up. If I was going to beat this drug thing, I had to leave.

I was wanted in St Louis and the police had told me to get out of town and never come back. That was where the Lord led me to go. I was arrested but I was given probation instead of prison. God blessed me in ways that I never imagined possible. He didn't just deliver me from my addiction, He put people in my life to help and encourage me. He keeps opening doors for me that seem locked shut.

He took a prison inmate and turned him into a prison chaplain. He took a bad check writer and made me a faith book writer. He took a person that had no hope and transformed him into a person who gives hope to the hopeless. The world saw a criminal, a zombie and a menace to society, but God saw something worth saving.

Psalm 121:3
He will not let you stumble;
the one who watches over you will not slumber.

About a month after I had left Chicago, I went back to take care of some unfinished business. My nephew, Chris, went with me. I ran into a couple of people that I used to hang with. I thought I had been clean long enough to be able to hang with them again and not use. That was a bad idea. I shot up with them. God reminded me of the day I sat on those church steps crying and begging Him to forgive me. I saw myself sitting there in the rain with drugs in my hand, listening to that sermon about the lost son. I heard God telling me again to leave Chicago. I started thinking about staying there that night and leaving the next day. Just then, Chris, who had been hanging with Ralph came back. He said, "Come on, Uncle Bub. Let's head back to St. Louis."

I believe that is why God had sent Chris to Chicago with me. We drove back to St. Louis that night. If I hadn't left that night, I would have fallen back into my old habits. I was in Chicago for one day and had stumbled, but God didn't let me fall. God uses different people to help keep you from falling. That night, He used Chris.

Psalm 121:4
Indeed, he who watches over Israel
never slumbers or sleeps.

I am so glad that God never sleeps or naps. There were so many times when He has watched over me day and night whether I was awake or asleep. One of those times was at my apartment, where I fell asleep on the couch after drinking. I woke up a few hours later and discovered that my apartment had been broken into. Some things had been taken, but God watched over me and I wasn't harmed.

Another time that God watched over me was when I overdosed on heroin in the bathroom in that same apartment one evening. I thank God that I wasn't alone that time. I don't know how long I had been out, but when I came to, I was lying on the couch. One of the guys who was there knew how to bring me out of it. Another time, I overdosed after shooting T's and Blues and God watched over me so that I may be revived once again.

When I was unconscious, I was at the mercy of the drug and its effect on my body. At any moment, my heart could've given out and there would've been nothing that I could've done about it. I would've peacefully slipped into this overdosed state and woke up on the other side of eternity. For reasons that only God knows, He didn't allow this to be the end of my story, when for so many of my friends, that was not the case.

I've passed out at least twice, and once I was so drunk, I fell asleep at a red light. I was on a main street about two blocks from the police station. I don't know how many times the light changed before I woke up. I just know that God watched over me.

Psalm 121: 5
The LORD himself watches over you!
The LORD stands beside you as your protective shade.

I remember walking to the corner store one day when I was about eight or nine years old. I knew God was with me, so I reached out for Him to hold my hand like my father did when we walked together. I felt His presence while we walked together, hand in hand. God has always been by my side, even when I was doing wrong. My father loved me. He didn't always agree with what I was doing or the life that I was living, but He never abandoned or gave up on me, even when I was strung out and acting crazy. That's how God is. He loves us unconditionally.

Psalm 121: 6
The sun will not harm you by day,
nor the moon at night.

God protects us from the dangers that we can see during the brightness of day, and from the dangers that we can't see because of the darkness of night. Our instructions are simply to listen to Him and follow His guidance. I've heard people say, "Something told me not to do that" or "Something told me not to go there." In fact, I've said it many times myself. I believe that "Something" is God and we tend to get ourselves in trouble when we don't listen to Him. For believers, we can't go where He told us not to go or do what He told us not to do. We have to always remember that God loves us and wants the best for us. If we trust and believe in Him, we don't have to worry about the day or the night, because God loves you.

Psalm 121: 7
The LORD keeps you from all harm
and watches over your life.

There were many times when I was robbed at gun point when I was going into or coming out of drug houses. I could have been killed during any of those instances, but God kept me. I could have died from any of the overdoses that I had, but God kept me. I was smoking crack with a young lady in a motel room one night. She said she was going to get some more drugs. I gave her some money and she left. Shortly after she left, "something" told me to get dressed and get out of there. When I got to my car I saw her coming down the street with two men. God kept me.

I got busted with heroin and cocaine one day. I had my syringe and cooker in my sock but they didn't find it. After they booked me, the officer asked if I had anything else on me. I said, "No." He told me that if he found something, he was going to hurt me and add what he found to my charges. He asked me again. Again, I said, "No". He found my syringe and cooker. I acted like I had forgotten that I had it and braced myself for a serious beat down. He didn't beat me up. Instead, he just shook his head and took me to lock up. God kept me.

Psalm 121:8
The LORD keeps watch over you as you come and go, both now and forever.

I know God is still watching over me. I have been blessed in ways that I know without a doubt, it had to be God. He leads me and guides me in the direction that He wants me to go. He showed me what my purpose is -- ministering to "the least of these".

This purpose has given me the positive outlet that I've always needed and it makes sense out of my chaotic life. Everything that I've endured, God is using to help save someone else. God was watching over me as a teenager when we were fighting with the local gangs in Chicago. He watched over me when I was getting high, getting robbed, getting locked up, getting shot or stabbed. God was watching over me through it all. When I speak in the prisons, He's watching over me. When I'm giving my testimony to a current addict or criminal, He's still watching over me while purifying my words so that I might say something that will give life, instead of take life.

I've been ministering to prisoners, ex-offenders, addicts and recovering addicts for more than 25 years. Tens of thousands of lives have been changed because of the ministry that God has given me. I want to be clear -- it is not me, it is God. I don't do this work alone. I have a team of dedicated people that work with me and I'm blessed with the opportunity to train other churches on how to do prison ministry.

Psalm 121

I don't know why Psalms 121 meant so much to my father or why he thought it was important that I read it so often. Maybe he wanted me to know that no matter how big a hill or mountain is, God can help me get over it. If I put my hand in God's hand, He will not let me fall. Maybe he wanted me to know that God never sleeps, and I can call on Him any time, even in the midnight hour. Maybe he wanted me to know that God has my back and will keep me and watch over me day and night. Maybe he wanted me to know that God will watch over me and protect me from evil. Maybe he wanted me to know that God will watch over me both now and forever. Whatever the reason was, it worked. It gave me what I needed in my fight against my addiction.

My father was a very wise man. In hindsight and with further enlightenment from God, I now realize the value of Psalm 121. He knew that God would restore all the years that the enemy stole from me; all 22 years, wandering through society as an addict, struggling to live out my purpose in life. Today, I share this gift with you.

ALSO BY BURTON BARR JR.

The Hoodlum Preacher:
I was Lost, Now I Am Found

Amazing Grace:
The Storm is Passing Over

He's Only a Prayer Away:
9 Examples of Praying Until Your
Breakthrough

God Still Loves You:
40 Reminders from God

121 (Documentary)

AVAILABLE AT
www.kobaltbooks.com

Burton Barr Jr.

CPSIA information can be obtained
at www.ICGtesting.com
Printed in the USA
BVHW080802010323
659310BV00002B/18